SHAPE UP, size down

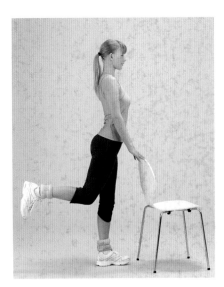

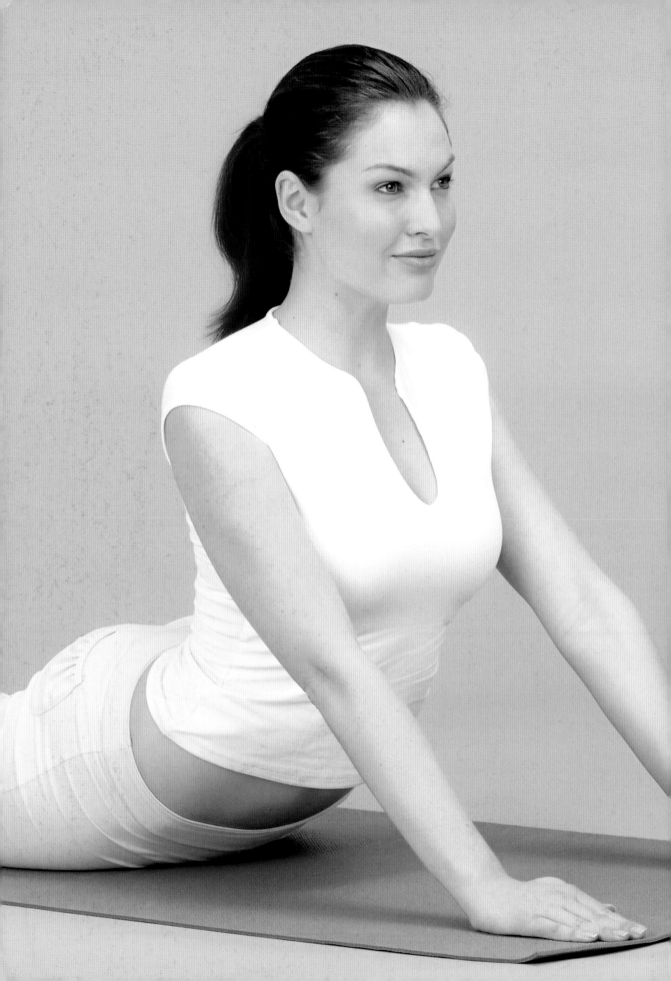

Sally Lewis

SHAPE UP, size down

Drop a dress size in only 4 weeks

hamlyn

An Hachette UK Company
www.hachette.co.uk

First published in Great Britain in 2009 by
Hamlyn, a division of Octopus Publishing Group Ltd
2–4 Heron Quays, London E14 4JP
www.octopusbooks.co.uk
www.octopusbooksusa.com

Distributed in the U.S. and Canada by Octopus Books USA:
c/o Hachette Book Group USA
237 Park Avenue, New York NY 10017

ISBN 978-0-600-61834-8

A CIP catalogue record for this book is available from the
British Library.

Printed and bound in China

10 9 8 7 6 5 4 3

Note

All reasonable care has been taken in the preparation of this book,
but the information it contains is not meant to take the place of
medical care under the direct supervision of a doctor. Before
making any changes in your health regime, always consult a doctor.
Any application of the ideas and information contained in this
book is at the reader's sole discretion and risk. Neither the author
nor the publisher will be responsible for any injury, loss, damages,
actions, proceedings, claims, demands, expenses and costs
(including legal costs or expenses) incurred in any way arising out
of following exercises in this book.

Contents

Introduction

This programme offers you the chance to create a new sexy, curvy, lighter you and at the same time it will increase your ability to deal with the stresses of modern living.

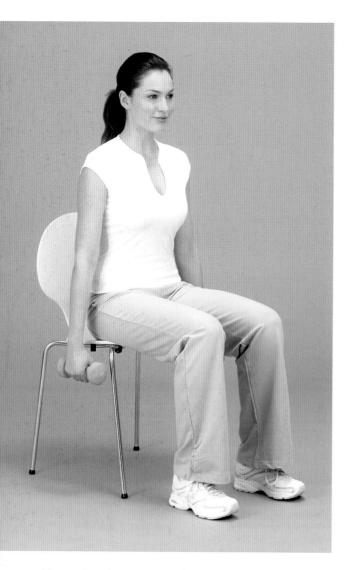

Above *Regular exercise is beneficial to your health and well-being. You will quickly discover that exercising gives you more energy and strength, while toning exercises will create a new leaner you.*

By incorporating the programme into your daily life, you will experience all the physical and psychological benefits that exercise has to offer (see pages 10–11), including weight loss, increased energy, a leaner, more toned body shape and the release of endorphins – chemicals within the brain that give you the 'feel-good' factor.

Establishing goals

One of the best ways to achieve the results you want is to set yourself goals, both short- and long-term ones. Write down your targets and place them somewhere you will see them regularly, such as on the fridge door. Keep your goals simple; it's very rewarding to tick off your successes as you achieve them and helps to keep you motivated. Once you have identified your aims, you will be surprised at how much better you feel about being in control of your life.

BENEFITS OF THE PROGRAMME

- Looking taller and slimmer
- Having tighter abdominal muscles
- Improving your body shape
- Feeling more motivated
- Relieving stress
- Improving your flexibility
- Boosting your general well-being

GOAL-SETTING

Be realistic: if you need to drop two dress sizes, realize that it will take longer than two or three weeks.

Be honest: if you have never exercised before, you are not going to be able to run a marathon within 12 weeks.

Identify what your real targets are.

Reward yourself when you reach a goal – book a massage, have a beauty treatment, buy a magazine or a new outfit (depending on your finances).

Be positive – if you really believe it will happen, it's much more likely to do so.

Why muscle loss and weight gain occur

It's not difficult to understand why we gain weight: usually it comes down to eating too much and having a sedentary lifestyle. However, many people do not realize that the ageing process also affects our weight. As we age we lose muscle mass – our muscles literally start to shrink. The loss of this lean muscle mass affects our metabolism, slowing it down, and as a result we gain weight and find it more difficult to lose it. Hormones also play an important role in affecting body weight after the age of 30 (see pages 10–11).

As we age, the number of calories that we need for energy decreases, because ageing promotes the replacement of muscle with fat. This is where this programme can help – not only by slowing down this process, but also by reverting it – by increasing the body's metabolism, toning and strengthening muscles and bones, helping you to lose weight and change body shape, while leaving you feeling healthier, energized, restored and motivated.

Calories

If you eat more than you require, you will add the excess as fat gain. Unless excess calories are burned up through exercise and movement, it is vital to eat the right types of food (such as vegetables and fruit) to prevent weight gain (see pages 14–15). Don't cut back drastically on your calorie intake, however, or your body will respond by conserving energy, making it even harder to lose those extra pounds.

Metabolic rate

Metabolism is the rate at which the body uses energy to support all the basic functions needed for life, energy and digestive processes. Basal Metabolic Rate (BMR) is the number of calories required for all essential bodily and chemical functions in a quiet and resting state. It is responsible for approximately 70 per cent of the calories burned in a day. Speeding up your metabolic rate by increasing your lean muscle mass will help you lose weight (see pages 12–13).

Apple or pear shape?

Our body shape is predominantly determined by the area where we store body fat and has a major influence on our health. Fat that is stored around the midriff area (including the stomach and bust) gives the appearance of a heavy torso with no waist definition and is known as an 'apple shape'. Fat that accumulates around the top of the thighs, bottom and hips gives rise to a 'pear shape'.

There is a lower risk of heart disease for pear-shaped women, and apple shapes are generally more at risk from diabetes, high blood pressure, strokes and breast cancer. It is healthier to be pear-shaped than apple-shaped because excess fat-deposits around the midriff tend to build up around the internal organs, such as the heart. After the menopause many women find that the fat from their bottoms, hips and thighs is redistributed to their waist, due to the decline in oestrogen produced by the ovaries.

Exercise

Finding time to exercise regularly is difficult for many people. But even simple changes can help, such as taking the stairs instead of the lift, parking the car a little further away from work or the shops, and walking at lunchtime. The programme requires just ten minutes of exercise at a time per day to make a difference (see pages 20–21) – so schedule it in your diary now!

ESTABLISHING YOUR SHAPE

Use the hip-to-waist ratio to determine your own body shape. Divide your waist measurement by your hip measurement: if the ratio is 0.8 or below, then you are pear-shaped; if it is greater than 0.8, you are apple-shaped.

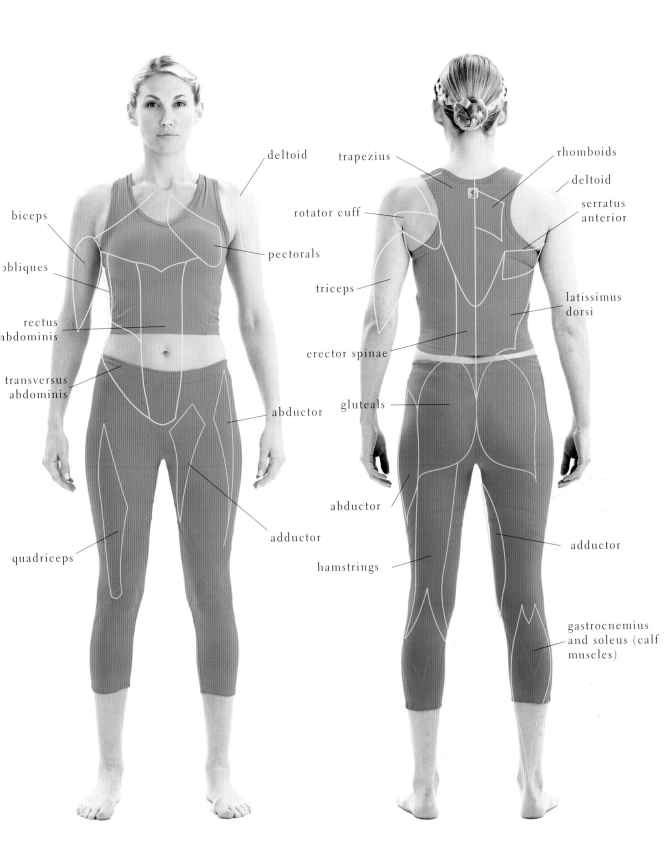

deltoid

biceps

obliques

rectus
abdominis

transversus
abdominis

pectorals

abductor

adductor

quadriceps

trapezius

rhomboids

deltoid

rotator cuff

serratus
anterior

triceps

latissimus
dorsi

erector spinae

gluteals

abductor

adductor

hamstrings

gastrocnemius
and soleus (calf
muscles)

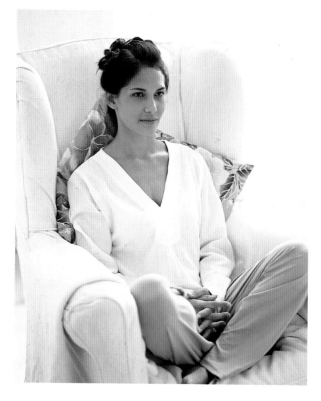

Above *Take time out of a busy day to practise deep-breathing and relaxation techniques to help you control your stress levels, and lower stress-related symptoms.*

LIFESTYLE ADVICE

- Get enough sleep to maintain healthy hormone levels.

- Take some exercise on a daily basis – the ten-minute routines from the programme are ideal.

- Eat a low-carbohydrate snack to increase the brain's levels of serotonin and reduce your cravings for sugar.

- Practise deep-breathing and relaxation techniques to control your stress levels and help lower your blood pressure and heart rate.

Harnessing hormones

If, no matter what you do, you can't seem to shift that excess weight gain, it may be that your body is attempting to sabotage your plans. Hormones are generally the key culprits in affecting body weight after the age of 30, and women are more susceptible than men because they often become hormonally out of balance, for dietary, lifestyle, emotional and physiological reasons. And the Western diet – with its processed foods, additives and chemicals – as well as stress and the frenetic pace of modern living can send our hormones spiralling out of control.

The effects of stress

Hormones are chemical messengers that create changes in our bodies. They vary on a daily basis, affecting our metabolism, mood and energy. Exercise also affects hormonal levels – they rapidly speed up, helping to burn calories and fat. However, the stress that we experience from rushing around, juggling home and family life, tension at work and tight schedules increases our levels of adrenaline and cortisol (a hormone connected to appetite). Excess stress over a period of time encourages the accumulation of 'stress fat', a build-up of fat just beneath the abdominal muscle, causing weight gain around the stomach area. This fat has been linked to high blood pressure, stroke, heart attacks and diabetes.

Sleep

Lack of sleep is another major factor that adversely affects hormone levels, in particular the amount of serotonin that we make. Serotonin controls our mood – it produces the 'feel-good' factor that we experience after exercise. If we experience a lack of serotonin, we become depressed; and the less serotonin we produce, the more we want to eat.

Insulin

Insulin is another hormone involved in weight gain. Produced by the pancreas, it is a blood-sugar regulator. The secretion of insulin rises rapidly after eating (especially carbohydrates) as blood-sugar levels increase. If the sugar is not quickly converted to energy, insulin converts the extra sugar to fat. That is a problem faced all too often by constant dieters and excess-carbohydrate eaters.

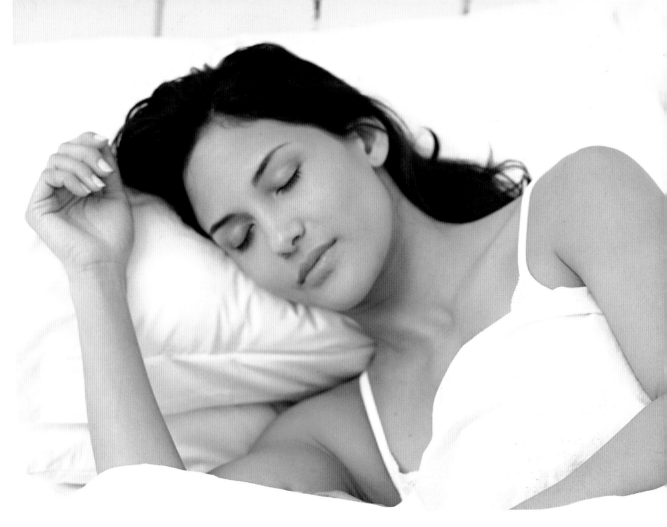

Menopause

Many women experience weight gain around the stomach and hips just before, during and after the menopause. It is often referred to as 'middle-age spread'. While hormone changes may be responsible for the gain, it is not irreversible or inevitable. Oestrogen levels do fall, but the real culprit is usually a combination of changing hormone levels, stress, excess toxins, a slowing down of the metabolism, an unhealthy diet and lack of exercise.

The benefits of diet and exercise

So what can you do to stop your hormones becoming so unsettled? Eating a nutritious diet is important (see pages 14–15). But another significant factor is exercise. Exercise not only burns calories (and, therefore, excess fat), but also helps to reduce stress levels, depression and anxiety, while improving overall health. You will feel and sleep better, deal with stress better and find that your mood improves.

Above *If you find getting to sleep difficult, give up tea, coffee, chocolate and cola at night since they are high in caffeine. Sleep is important in maintaining optimum health and well-being.*

To get real benefits you need to exercise on a daily basis. Lacking time is a common excuse, but the programme's unique ten-minute routines – ideally done three times a day – ensure that even the busiest people can find time to introduce daily exercise into their lives and get great results. This will leave you feeling good and will have a positive impact on your health and well-being.

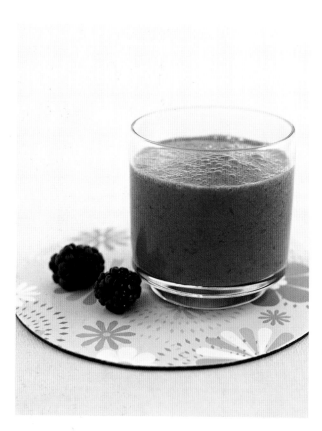

Above *Fresh fruit and vegetable juices are delicious, easy to digest and offer real health benefits.*

QUIZ YOURSELF

- Do you feel tired and lethargic?
- Do you wake up after eight hours' sleep and still have to drag yourself out of bed?
- Do you avoid exercise because you simply haven't the energy?

If you answered 'Yes' to any of these questions, the chances are that your metabolism needs boosting. The programme offers you the opportunity to revitalize your metabolism naturally, providing you with the energy to meet the challenges of modern living.

Fuelling your metabolism

Metabolism is the amount of energy (calories) that your body needs on a daily basis to support all the functions required for life, energy and digestive processes. Sleeping, eating, drinking and thinking all require energy, so calories are constantly being used up. Metabolism varies hugely from person to person: some people can eat like a horse and remain skinny, while others only have to look at a biscuit to pile on the pounds – this is down to their metabolic rate. Other factors include your gender, age and ratio of muscle to fat.

As you age, your body's metabolism naturally slows down, often resulting in weight gain and general lethargy. Your natural functions (such as digestion) also slow down. However, by boosting your metabolism through exercise and good nutrition you can reverse these effects, encouraging your body to use up stored body fat and increase your digestion and mental ability, leaving you feeling refreshed.

Increasing your BMR

The number of calories you burn each day is affected by how much you exercise, the amount of muscle and fat you have and your own Basal Metabolic Rate – the speed at which you burn calories while 'at rest'. Although you may have inherited your BMR, you can also change it through exercise and good nutrition (see pages 8–9).

Toned muscles

Tone your muscles – toned muscles boost your metabolism and muscles use more energy than fat. The rate at which your body burns calories is partly determined by the amount of muscle you have. The more muscle, the higher your metabolic rate. A 20-year-old burns more calories than a 70-year-old because he or she has more muscle mass. The programme uses toning and resistance exercises to build muscle mass and speed up metabolism. Any form of aerobic exercise – such as jogging, running, cycling or swimming – will boost your metabolism, and simply being more energetic every day will keep it that way. Muscle mass uses up 30–50 calories per day, compared with just two calories a day for fat. And the more muscle you have, the higher your metabolic rate.

QUICK WAYS TO BOOST YOUR METABOLISM

- Eat breakfast.
- Eat smaller meals more frequently – aim for four or five throughout the day.
- Drink plenty of water: at least eight glasses a day.
- Get enough vitamin B; try a vitamin B-complex supplement, if necessary.
- Juice up – raw vegetables and fruit are easily digested and ensure an optimum supply of vitamins and minerals.
- Eat spices: add some chillies to your food.
- Drink green tea, which contains antioxidants that speed up your metabolism.
- Have a sauna (health conditions permitting), as heat increases your metabolic rate.
- Build muscle with toning/resistance exercises at least three times per week.
- Get some aerobic exercise, such as a brisk walk, for 20 minutes a day.

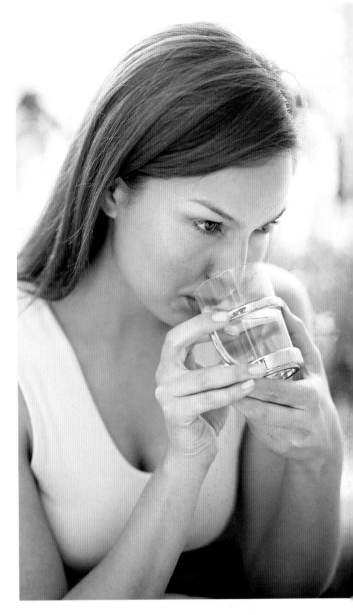

Above *Drinking 6–8 glasses of water a day will help to keep you hydrated, boosting your metabolism by flushing out the toxins that can make it sluggish.*

Calorie-counting

Eating too many calories will ultimately result in weight gain, but eating fewer than 1,000 calories a day will also affect your weight. Nutritionists have discovered that the metabolism slows down when fewer calories are consumed. The body holds on to fat reserves, making weight loss harder to achieve, because it believes it is in starvation mode and retains any excess fat, which has an adverse effect on energy levels. On average a women requires 2000 calories a day, a man 2,500. You need to eat approximately 500 calories less a day to lose weight. You can burn up extra calories by increasing the amount of muscle in your body by exercising using weights.

Eat right

Understanding what foods we need to eat in order to lose weight is a key factor in improving our figures and our health.

The body is a complex machine requiring the correct nutritional balance to run efficiently. The main food groups that we depend on are carbohydrates, protein, fats, vitamins and minerals, each of which has a specific role to play.

Food groups explained

Complex carbohydrates These 'starchy' foods are high in fibre and are converted into glucose, a form of sugar used by the body to give you energy. Brown rice, brown pasta, wholemeal bread, potatoes, lentils and beans, oats and wholegrain cereals are good examples.

Below *All fresh fruit and vegetables are high in vitamins and minerals, and low in calories. Try to ensure you eat as wide a range as possible.*

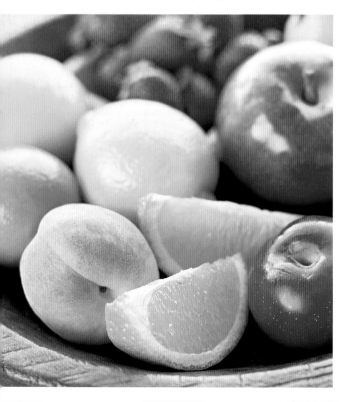

Protein Protein is essential for growth and repair of the body and, importantly, for building and repairing muscle. The more muscle we have, the more calories we burn. Protein-rich foods include chicken, lean meat, fish, tofu, eggs, pulses and milk. However, choose lean meat and cut off any excess fat; and grill or oven-cook it, rather than frying it. Protein should provide no more than 15 per cent of your daily calorie consumption.

DIETARY ESSENTIALS

- Eat a balance of protein and complex carbohydrates every day.

- Consume a least five portions of fruit and vegetables a day.

- Women need 100 g (3½ oz) of protein in their diet per day; men need 150 g (5 oz).

ENERGY-BOOSTING FOODS

Oats, muesli, nuts and seeds, fish and poultry, baked potatoes, fruit and vegetables, natural fruit juice, water, extra-virgin organic olive oil

ENERGY-DEPLETING FOODS

Caffeine, refined sugar, hydrogenated fats (e.g. pies and sausage rolls), crisps, white bread, carbonated drinks, processed food

Fats A great source of energy, fats provide twice as many calories as carbohydrates or protein and are often neglected, for fear of weight gain. Avoid saturated fats; choose polyunsaturated and monounsaturated fats, such as virgin olive oil, safflower, sunflower and rapeseed oil, nuts, seeds and oily fish, for beneficial energy levels.

Vitamins and minerals These are essential to maintain the body's metabolic functions. The body manufactures a few vitamins and minerals itself, but most have to be found in the food we eat, including meat, cereals, fish, fruit, vegetables, nuts, eggs and dairy produce.

The vitality diet

A simple way to boost your metabolism is to eat for energy. Vitamin B is often lacking in the diets of those who feel lethargic, and the best sources are fruit, raw vegetables, wheat germ, seeds and nuts, chicken, meat, fish, eggs and dairy products. Try juicing raw vegetables or fruit for a rich supply of vitamins and minerals.

The key for optimum energy is to maintain your blood sugar at a constant level, so eating small, regular meals is preferable to two or three large meals. Cutting back on caffeine, processed foods, sugar and saturated fats, and replacing them with nutritious options, will increase energy levels. Complex carbohydrates such as brown bread, brown rice, brown pasta, vegetables, fruit and lean protein are the best foods to eat.

Stress adversely affects metabolism. Eating well will help your adrenal glands, which among other functions top up energy levels and help the body deal with stress, to function properly. Prolonged stress will deplete vital sources of minerals such as zinc; magnesium, copper, sodium and potassium.

Another key is breakfast, which prepares your body for the day ahead. Make sure you drink enough water, as this is vital to keep your body running efficiently.

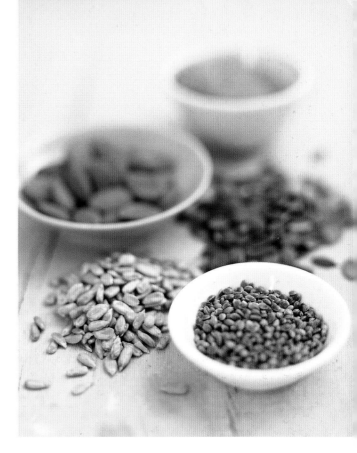

Above *Nuts and seeds provide unsaturated, healthy fats, known as essential fatty acids, and are a good source of protein, fibre and essential vitamins.*

An ideal daily diet

Choose one suggestion from each section below:

Breakfast Complex carbohydrates: cereal or muesli with semi-skimmed or skimmed milk, topped with berries or natural yoghurt; or poached eggs on wholemeal toast; or porridge with a little honey.

Lunch Rice with lean chicken or fish and salad; or a wholemeal roll filled with a lean source of protein and salad; or a jacket potato and tuna; or avocado and chicken salad.

Dinner Salmon with vegetables and rice; or chicken with stir-fried vegetables; or fish kebabs with wild rice; or pork fillet with new potatoes and vegetables.

Snacks Eat two a day: a banana; oatcakes with peanut butter; rice cakes and cheese; an apple or a handful of grapes; a small handful of nuts and seeds.

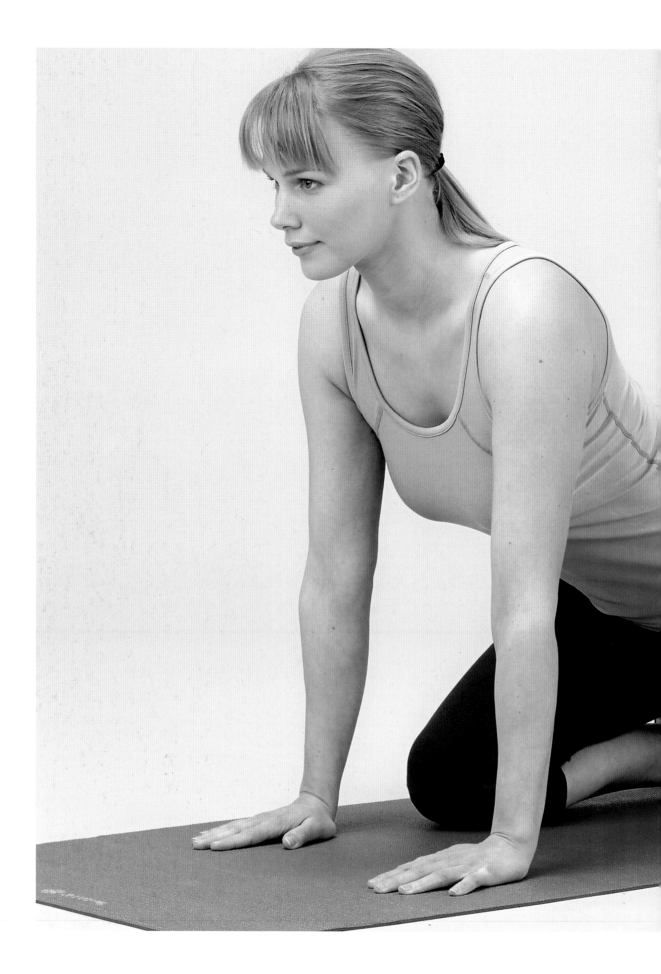

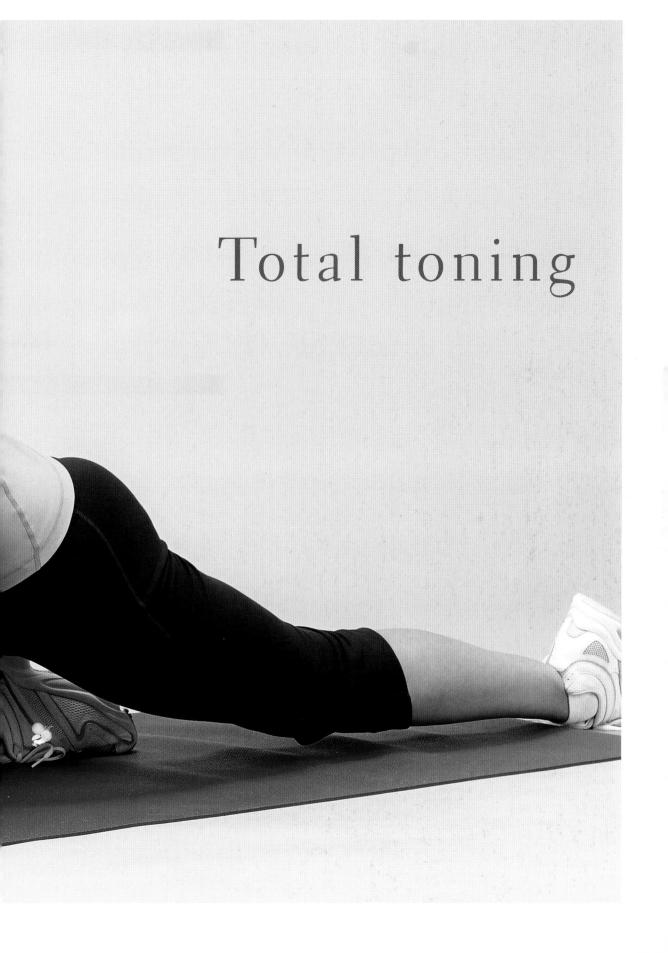

Total toning

The right combination

The programme aims to **tone all of your body**, but easily adapts to your needs if you wish to work on specific areas, such as your shoulders or core muscles.

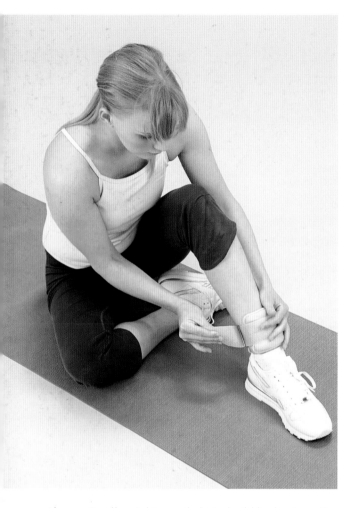

Above *Small weights can help to build body strength, improving posture and making daily tasks easier.*

It is important to remember that if you tone the whole of your body, it will emphasize your shape and physique. A lean body with sculpted shoulders and arms will encourage you to stand taller and will automatically make you look slimmer; and a strong core will ensure improved posture and a leaner figure.

As you tone your muscles you will increase your metabolism, which will help you burn fat faster and lose weight. Toning exercises help to release stress from the body, keeping you fitter, stronger and in better general health.

Equipment

The programme does not require expensive equipment. For the arms, shoulders, chest and back exercises you can use hand dumb-bells with a weight range of 0.5–2 kg (1–5 lb) upwards. If you don't want to go to the expense of hand weights, two cans of food or two filled water bottles will suffice. Wrap-around ankle weights can be used to increase the intensity of the exercise.

If this is the first time you have exercised, or you are returning to exercise after a long break, you may not need to use hand or ankle weights at all, or may only feel comfortable with 500 g (1 lb) weights. Gradually challenge your muscles by increasing the weights over the weeks. A Swiss ball (also known as a body ball, gym ball or fitness ball) is another useful tool if you wish to work harder and perform some of the advanced exercises. It should be burst-resistant and able to take at least 300 kg (660 lb) in weight. Make sure you use the correct size for your height – when you sit on the ball, your knees should be slightly lower than your hips. Swiss balls come in four diameters: 45 (18 in) 55 (22 in), 65 (26 in) and 75 cm (30 in). The recommended height–ball-size ratio is as follows:

- **152 cm (5 ft) or less:** 45 cm
- **155–167 cm (5 ft 1 in–5 ft 6 in):** 55 cm
- **170–185 cm (5 ft 7 in–6 ft 1 in):** 65 cm
- **188 cm (6 ft 2 in) or above:** 75 cm

An exercise mat is useful, but not essential (you can use a towel instead).

Other types of exercise

You need to include a combination of exercises for the best results. These include cardiovascular work, resistance work and flexibility (enabling the muscles to stretch and relax). It is vital to warm up and cool down before and after any exercise (see pages 26–29).

Cardiovascular exercise

Any form of exercise that increases your heart rate and makes you out of breath is aerobic exercise, which helps to build your stamina. Running, cycling, swimming, mini-trampolining, skipping, dancing, stepping, jogging and even brisk walking are suitable aerobic work.

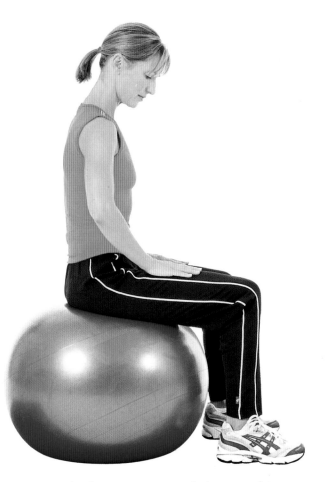

Above *Check your posture regularly, even when sitting and remember to engage your core muscles before you begin exercising.*

EXERCISE ADVICE

- Toning exercises targeted at specific areas bring about great results, but it is much more beneficial to concentrate on the body as a whole.

- Aim to work out for 30 minutes at least three times per week, by selecting three of the ten-minute routines from the programme (see pages 20–21 and 114–125).

- Try to add one to three 20-minute aerobic sessions to your exercise programme per week.

Resistance work

Resistance exercises work on specific parts of the body where the muscles apply force to an external resistance. You can either use loose weights, gym equipment, water bottles or your own body weight to add resistance to the muscles. These exercises will help to tone and shape your body as well as helping to burn fat; increasing overall lean muscle mass by using up calories, the muscles convert fat into energy, and at the same time boosting your metabolism. Resistance training will also help build strong bones, and improves bone density helping to guard against osteoporosis. It also has a positive effect on blood pressure and body fat, and can greatly reduce a number of health risks including diabetes and heart disease. A step, chair or fitness ball will also bring a new dimension to your workout and make the exercise more effective.

Planning your programme

The unique ten-minute routines of the programme are devised to work on specific areas of the body; using both the upper- and lower-body routines, you can **reshape your body and size down within weeks**. There are a number of factors to take into account.

How often?

You need to do the exercises for at least 30 minutes a minimum of three times per week – and preferably six times, as in the Four-Week Plan on pages 114–125, making sure that you perform all of the repetitions mentioned in the text. Once you start to see improvements, you can increase the number of repetitions for each exercise.

It is best to work on different muscle groups at a time and make sure they have a rest in between – for example, work on your upper body one day and your lower body the next, then go back to your upper body. The Four-Week Plan has already done this for you.

Putting it into practice

The most common excuse for not doing exercise is the time it takes. That's why the programme is so great – anyone can find just ten minutes at a time. If you can manage three ten-minute sessions a day for six days, plus up to three 20-minute aerobic exercise sessions each week, for the next four weeks, you will soon see a difference. If you decide to do your own ten-minute routines, keep a record of the exercises you select, so that you work all the areas of your body.

Decide when you can exercise each day and schedule it into your diary – treat it as you would a business meeting or social occasion. Pick a time to suit your lifestyle, whether that's first thing in the morning (boosting your metabolism for the day) or in the late afternoon/early evening (when you should be at your most flexible).

Don't forget that to shape up and size down successfully, you need to combine your exercise with healthy eating (see pages 14–15) to deal with the excess flab you may have around your middle.

Below *You will quickly discover that exercising gives you more energy and gradually it will become part of your everyday routine and way of life.*

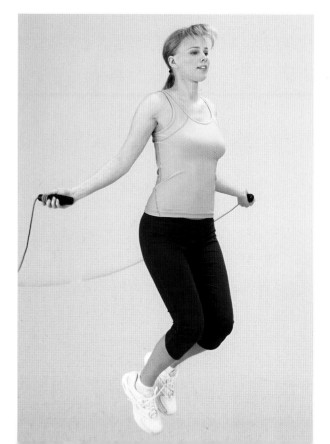

Warming up

It is important to spend a few minutes getting the muscles and joints ready for your workout, increasing your heart rate and pumping your blood around your body. Brisk walking, jogging, mini-trampolining, cycling and skipping all increase your body temperature. Add a few stretches, too – the side, triceps, hamstring and calf stretches on pages 26–27 are ideal.

Cooling down

Just as you have prepared your body for exercise, so you need to cool it down afterwards. Try to complete all the stretches on pages 28–29.

The exercises

There are two stages to the programme: the beginners' version (the main exercise in each case) and sometimes an advanced version (called 'Really work it!'). Start with the beginner's versions, even if you are returning to exercise after a period off. Then you can incorporate the advanced exercises, aiming for your long-term goals.

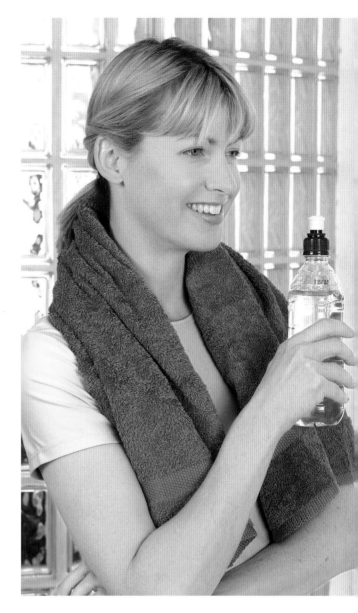

Above *Get into the habit of reaching for the water bottle. You should drink water before, during and after exercise to replace any lost fluids.*

PROGRAMME ADVICE

- Ideally, follow the Four-Week Plan on pages 114–125.

- Alternatively, write down your own programme in chart form and stick to it for a week, making sure you choose exercises from each section.

- Remember to drink water before, during and after your workout.

- Concentrate on each exercise as you perform it.

- Give yourself a posture check every few hours (see pages 24–25).

- Tell yourself that in just four weeks you can change your life and body shape, and boost your confidence.

Before you begin

The programme is **safe and easy** to follow. It allows you to make the decisions as to when and where you exercise, although there are various points to bear in mind before you begin. As with any exercise regime, it is a good idea to consult your doctor or other health professional before you begin.

When to exercise

It doesn't matter what time of day you exercise – it comes down to working out how you can fit it into your day. Among some professionals, exercising in the morning is considered to raise the metabolic rate and keep it elevated for longer throughout the day; however, some people prefer exercising between 4 and 7 p.m. when the body has warmed up and is more flexible. Consistency is the key; while you may alter the times in the day when you exercise, you need to make sure you schedule in the right number of times each week: three ten-minute sessions, six times per week.

How to exercise

Muscles that have not been worked before or for a long time tire quickly, so don't be tempted to do too much too soon or you may put yourself off exercising. It can often be 24 hours after you have exercised that your muscles ache.

If any exercises are painful, check that you are performing them correctly, for you may be using too much weight. Keep a note of how many exercises you perform and the numbers of repetitions for each exercise as you go along. It is easy to build in more repetitions and sets and, if appropriate, increase your weights as you find the exercises getting easier, the fitter you become. Once you feel comfortable working on the beginner's versions, move on to the advanced versions. Should you find yourself feeling dizzy or light-headed

Below *Keep a chart of your exercise sessions. Record the exercises you do and the number of repetitions; this way you will be able to see how you are progressing.*

Right *Posture is important, even when stretching. Try to make sure you have a mirror available so you can check your posture at different times.*

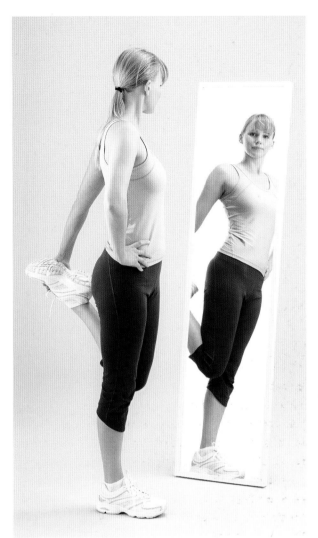

at any time, stop exercising and wait for it to pass; if it happens again, consult your doctor. Always warm up and cool down (see pages 26–29) to help protect you from injury.

Other considerations

Your workout area should be warm, but not hot, and have non-slip flooring. Wear appropriate clothing (and footwear, if necessary): a T-shirt, shorts or leggings, with a good support or sports bra; plus a pair of suitable trainers. Always have some water available and eat something within one hour of completing your exercise programme. However, is advisable not to eat two hours before you start to exercise. Posture (see pages 24–25) is all-important when you exercise, so try and exercise in front of a mirror. Concentrate on each exercise and do not perform it too quickly. Research shows that when you concentrate on the muscles you are using, they will work harder, producing better results.

Motivation

You may feel reluctant to start exercising, even though you know it is good for you; that you have insufficient time; or that you don't have the right equipment or gym membership to exercise properly. But this programme dispels all of this: you can get results in the privacy of your own home, with little or no equipment. Once you feel and see the changes, you will feel motivated and energized, which will improve your overall well-being.

There are some simple ways that you can get and stay motivated, one of those is to have a schedule. The programme gives you maximum help as the exercises have been selected into ten minute routines for you. All you have to do is follow through the four-week plan on pages 114–125. It will help you to stay motivated if you have someone to exercise with, so ask a friend to join you. Plan your exercise sessions together and write them in your diaries, that way you are less likely to find an excuse. Focus on what you want to achieve, whether it is dropping a dress size or losing a few kilos; make a note of your goals and record your progress.

MOTIVATIONAL ADVICE

- Exercise with a friend.
- Play some inspirational music.
- Set a goal, such as dropping a dress size – and buy a dress one size smaller now!
- Mark each exercise session on your calendar.
- Plan ahead.
- Keep a record of your progress.

Posture and balance

Balance of the mind, body and spirit is important if you are **to maintain good health**, yet it is constantly challenged by the stresses of modern living.

For our bodies to function efficiently and provide us with the energy we need to feel good about ourselves, they have to adapt to the onslaught of environmental, physical and physiological changes that beset us. Good nutrition, sleep, exercise and relaxation are imperative to help us achieve a sense of well-being.

Below *Good posture will make you look taller and leaner and help to prevent back problems.*

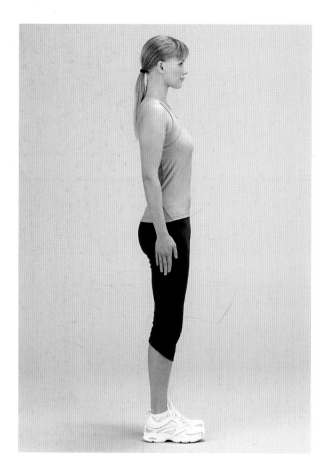

Posture

We all know what posture is – it's what we forget about when sitting at our desks or slumped in a chair watching television. But it is vital to have correct posture, for no amount of exercise can alter your body shape if your posture is incorrect. Poor posture affects us in many ways: it creates tension in the shoulders, contributes to lower back pain, lack of energy, bad circulation and general muscle aches and pains; it affects our breathing and our energy. Posture also has a huge impact on our muscle tone: bad posture leads to tight, shortened muscles and muscle imbalance, and there may be an uneven distribution of muscle tone, creating a distorted body shape. Being aware of good posture while exercising goes a long way to achieving the results you want.

Realigning the body through good posture can go a long way to redressing the problems we have created,

WHAT IS GOOD STANDING POSTURE?

- There should be a straight line through your ears, shoulders, hips, knees and ankles.
- Hold your head up, with your chin in.
- Keep your shoulders drawn back and down.
- Pull in your tummy, but do not arch your back or tip your pelvis.

encouraging the muscles to stretch and lengthen, releasing tension, toxins and waste and encouraging blood to flow freely around the body. When we exercise it is important to be aware of posture at all times. The benefits of good posture are numerous:

- The body suffers from less muscular pain (for example, in the lower back or shoulders).
- The skeleton moves more efficiently.
- Muscle function improves.
- The body's range of motion increases.
- The circulation improves.
- A slimmer, longer appearance is created.
- Confidence increases.
- Breathing is more efficient.

Balance

Posture and balance are interconnected. Good balance keeps you mobile and gives you energy and strength; as you get older it also helps to protect you from injuries and falls. If you have good posture, your balance is probably good too – although you can have excellent balance at the expense of posture. Hand in hand, balance and posture provide you with leaner, longer muscles, defining your body shape and adding elegance; they also strengthen the mind, creating inner harmony and strength.

It is worth practising positions that challenge your sense of balance. Become aware of how much you have to concentrate to keep your body from moving. This focuses the mind and encourages deeper breathing, fuelling the cells with oxygen; it also centres the body's core muscles (including the back and stomach muscles), causing them to engage and making you more aware of them.

Balancing exercise

Stand with your feet hip-width apart, hands by your sides, shoulders drawn back and down and chin lifted. Breathe in and draw your belly button back to your spine. Breathe out as you place your right foot on the inside left thigh, above your left knee, turning your right knee out to a 45-degree angle. Lift your arms above your head, palms together. Hold for five to ten seconds. Slowly lower your right foot to the floor and your arms back to your sides. Repeat on the other leg.

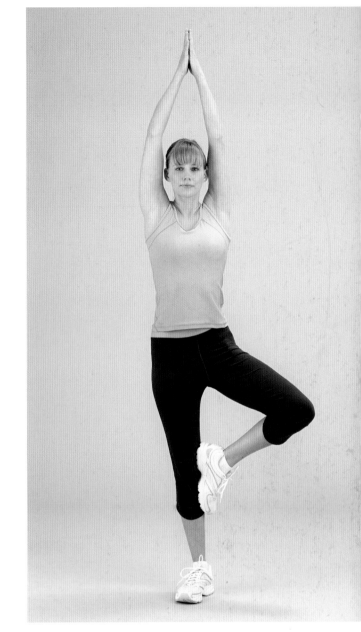

Above *Balance is essential for keeping you healthy and mobile, enabling you to move freely whilst increasing your energy and strength.*

Warm up

As we have seen, before commencing your exercise routine **it is vital to spend a few minutes stretching** the muscles and getting the joints ready for your workout, so try these simple stretches.

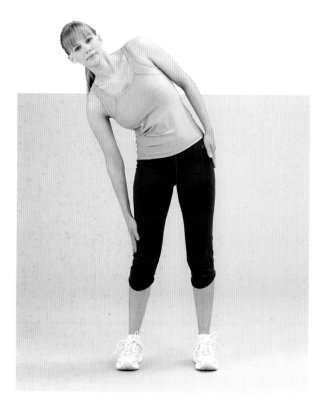

△ Side stretch

Stand with your feet facing forward, hip-width apart, and your arms resting down each side of your body. Breathe out and slide your right hand down the right side of your leg, letting your head drop over to the right shoulder. Stretch your fingers downwards, and make sure you pull in your abdominals to maximize the stretch. Breathe in and return to the starting position. Repeat down the left-hand side.

▽ Triceps stretch

Stand with your feet hip-width apart, toes pointing forwards and a slight bend in your knees. Lift your right arm up above your head, then bend the elbow and put the lower arm and hand behind your head; push the fingers of your right hand between your shoulder blades. Place your left arm across the top of your head and your fingers round the right elbow. As you reach with your right hand between your shoulder blades, push gently on the right arm with your left hand. Hold for a count of ten seconds and then release both arms. Repeat on the left side.

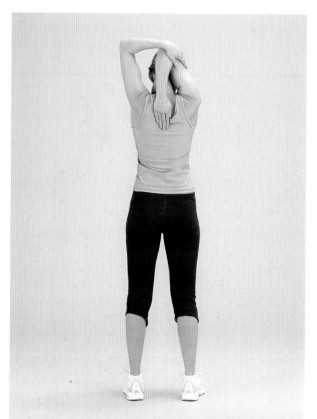

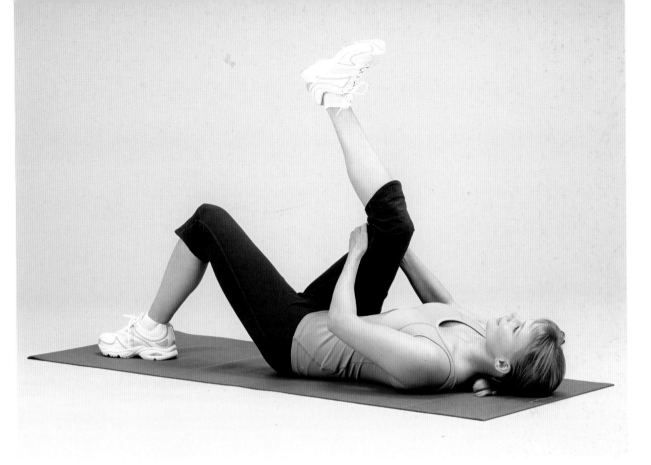

△ Hamstring stretch

Lie on your back on the mat with your feet hip-width apart. Both knees should be bent, with the feet flat on the floor. Slide your hands under your right thigh and lift your right leg straight up, with the sole of the foot facing the ceiling. The right knee should remain slightly bent. Gently pull your right thigh towards your chest. Hold for 15 seconds. Repeat on the left side.

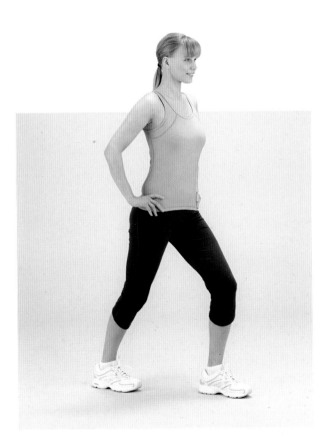

◁ Calf stretch

Step forward with your left foot and place both hands on your hips. Your hips, shoulders and feet should all be facing forward. Keeping both heels on the ground, bend your left knee slowly and feel the stretch; keep the right leg straight. Hold for a count of ten seconds. Repeat on the other side. You can also do this using a wall, stand facing a wall approximately 1 m (3 ft) away, step forward with your left foot and place both hands on the wall in front of you, elbows slightly bent. Continue with the stretch as above.

Cool down

In the same way that you prepared your body for exercise, so you need to **cool it down afterwards**. Try to do all the stretches described here.

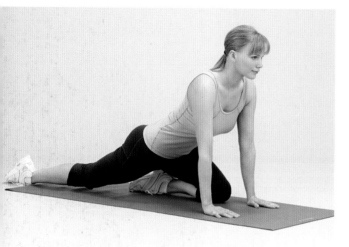

▽ Quad stretch

Stand with your feet hip-width apart and arms by your sides. Bend your right knee and lift the foot behind you. Grasp the right foot with your right arm and pull the heel towards your bottom, at the same time gently tilting the pelvis forward, keeping the knees in line. Release the left hand out to the side at shoulder height or extend it straight up to the ceiling, whichever you find easiest to retain your balance. You can hold on to a wall or the back of a chair for support if you need to. Repeat on the other side.

△ Hip flexor

Kneel on the mat with your arms down by your sides and your hands flat on the floor. Extend your right leg out behind you and press your bottom and hips down gently towards the floor. Hold for a count of 5 and then gently slide the right leg back in. Repeat on the left side.

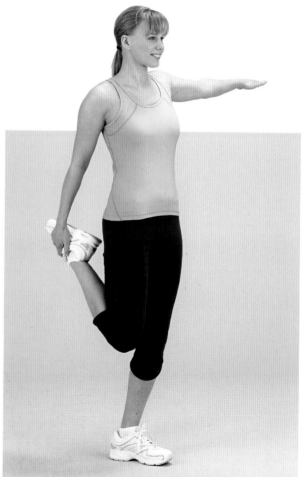

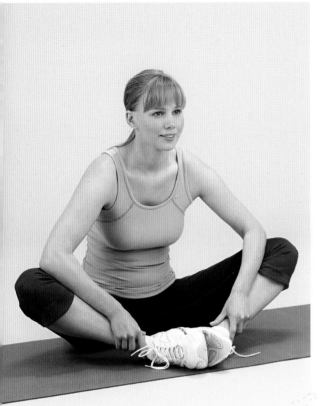

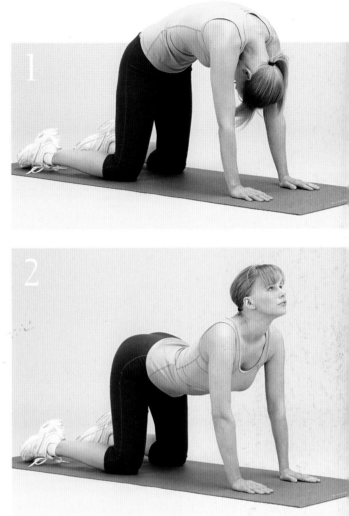

△ Inner-thigh stretch

Sit on the mat, with your back straight and the soles of your feet together. Taking hold of your feet with your hands, gently drop the knees out to the sides as you breathe out. Press the knees gently down with your elbows, then hold the stretch for ten seconds. Do not bounce the stretch.

△ Cat stretch

1 Kneel on all fours on the mat, with your legs hip-width apart. Your knees should be directly under your hips, and your hands under your shoulders. Breathe in as you pull up your abdominal muscles and pelvic-floor muscle and draw your belly button in towards your spine. Keep drawing your spine upwards as you arch your back, keeping your head down and your chin tucked under.

2 Breathe out as you reverse the arch by pressing down through your back and lifting your head and chin. Pull your shoulders back and down. Do four complete stretches.

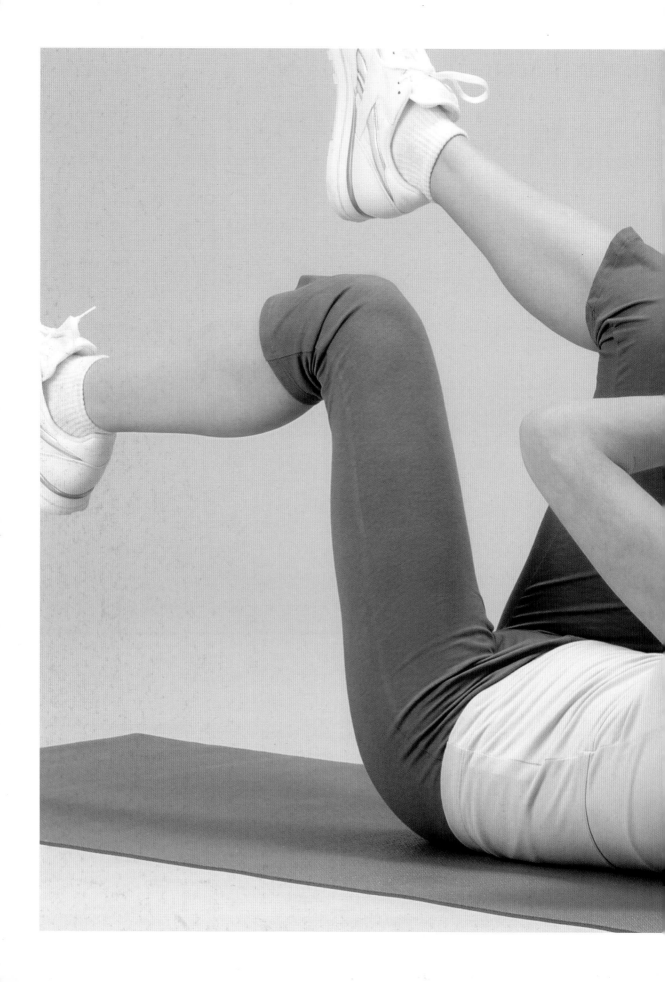

Getting a grip
on love handles

stomach CRUNCH

The aim of this exercise is to work on the major stomach muscles, both at the front and side of the stomach. You will tone and tighten the oblique externus abdominis and oblique internus abdominis muscles, giving you **a flatter, toned tummy**.

TRAINER TIP

Make sure you do not strain your neck by pulling on your head with your hands.

1 Lie on your back with your knees bent and hip-width apart, feet flat on the floor. Put your fingertips on each side of your head.

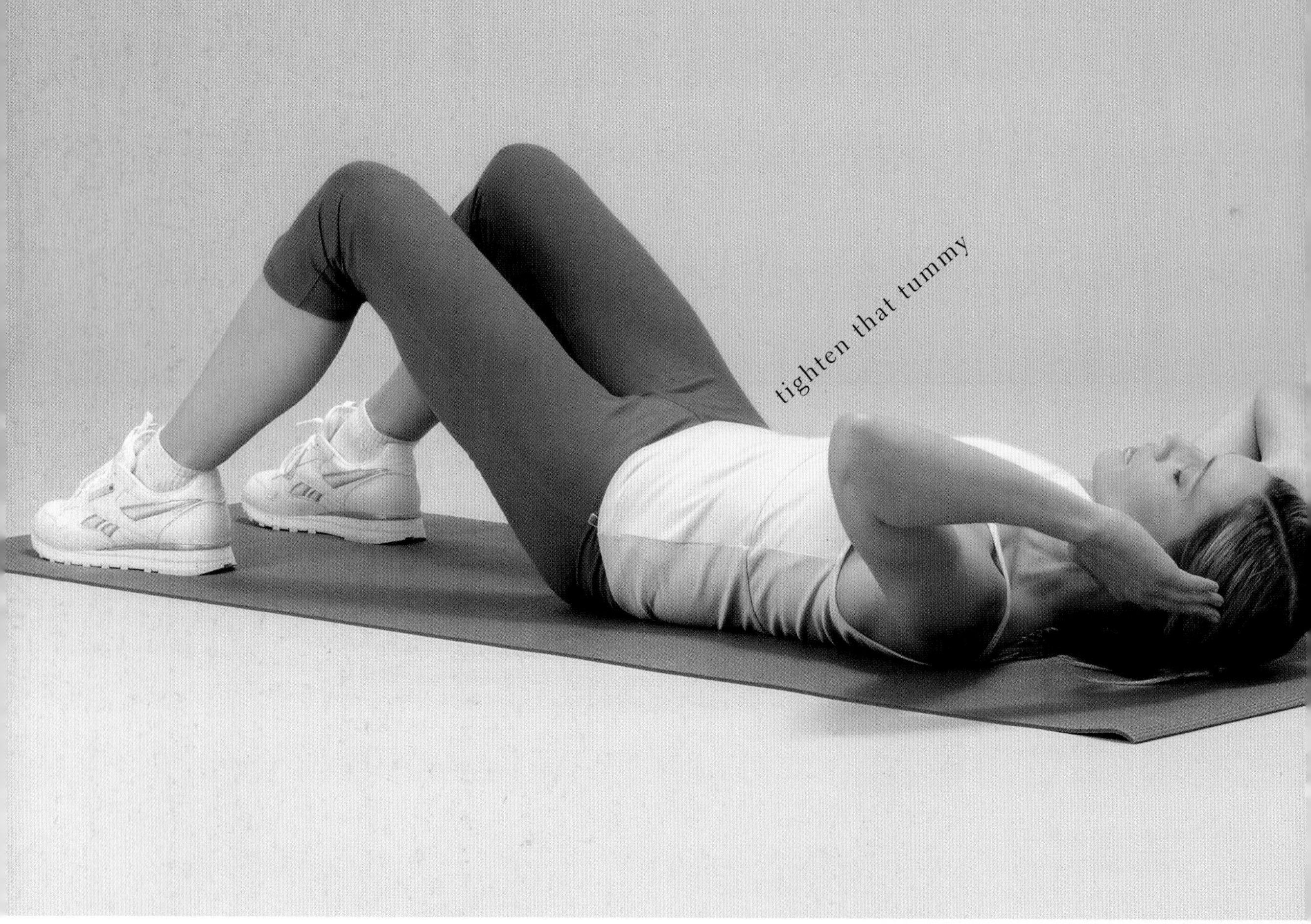

tighten that tummy

2 Breathe out as you tense your abdominal muscles and lift your head and shoulders off the floor. Keep your chin lifted, so that there is a space between it and your chest. Hold for a count of two. Breathe in as you lower slowly back down. Aim for 16 crunches.

REALLY WORK IT!

Perform this exercise with a Swiss ball once you feel able to manage at least three sets of the basic crunch. Lie backwards on the ball, with it resting on your lower back. Place your fingertips on each side of your head.

Breathe out as you tense your abdominal muscles and lift your head and shoulders, crunching forward. Hold the contraction for two seconds, then slowly breathe in and relax back to the starting position. Aim for 16 crunches.

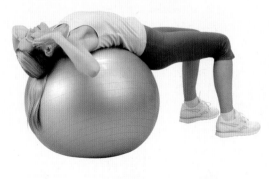

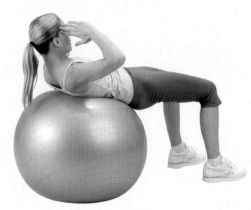

the PLANK

This exercise focuses on developing the small, deep muscles in the stomach (the transverse abdominis) and the muscle running up the side of the spine. It will support your back, giving you **good posture and a firm tummy**, and help to reduce or prevent back pain.

1 Lie flat on the floor on your stomach. Make a fist with each hand, then rest your upper body weight on your elbows, with your fists just in front of your shoulders. Your body and legs should be in a straight line.

2 Lift your body up onto your elbows and toes. Pull up your pelvic floor and stomach muscles and hold. Ensure that your back is in a straight line – this may mean you have to tip your pelvis up a little, but be careful not to lift your hips too high. Hold the position for ten seconds. Your aim is to be able to hold for one minute eventually. Lower back down to the floor. Rest for 30 seconds, then repeat four more times.

keep it straight

REALLY WORK IT!

If you can hold the basic position five times for a minute each, move on to this version. Lie flat on the floor as before, with your hands making fists. Lift your body up onto your elbows and toes, then extend your right leg out behind you and hold for 15 seconds.

Lower it, then lift the left leg and hold for 15 seconds. Your aim is to hold for one minute eventually. Lower back down to the floor. Repeat on both legs four more times.

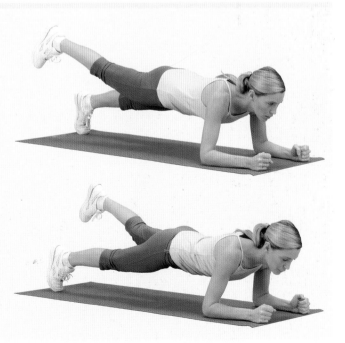

heel TOUCH

The heel touch works all of the rectus abdominis muscle, but you will feel it first in the lower part of your stomach. It is a very effective move that helps to flatten the stomach.

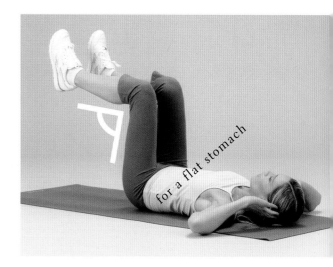

for a flat stomach

1 Lie on your back with your arms by your sides. Bend your knees and lift them so that they are perpendicular to the floor.

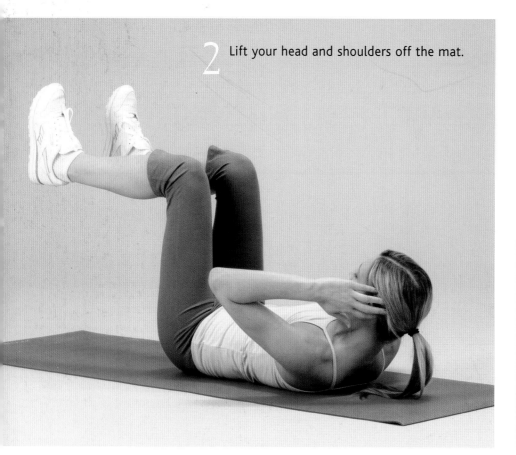

2 Lift your head and shoulders off the mat.

TRAINER TIP

Keep your back pressed down as you lower and raise your legs, by concentrating on your abdominals.

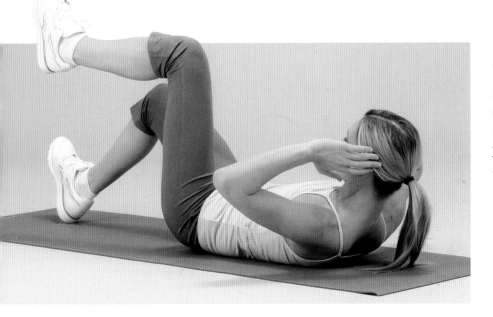

3 Slowly lower the left leg to the floor with the heel leading, letting the heel tap the floor, then lift it back up to the starting position. Keep your lower back pressed into the floor.

4 Repeat with the right leg. If you need to make this easier, bend your knees more and do not lower your heels down so far. Aim for 16 repetitions.

reverse CURL

This exercise tones and strengthens the major stomach muscles, but **targets the lower abdominal muscles** by bringing the pelvis towards the chest. You may find this challenging to begin with, but as your stomach muscles strengthen you will be able to perform more repetitions.

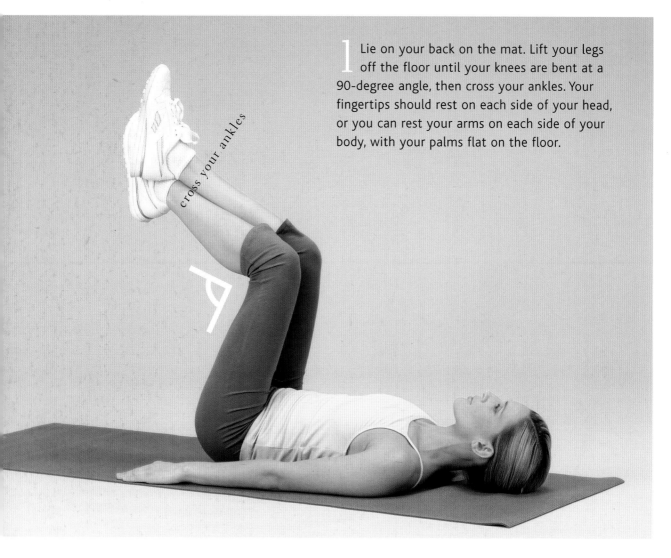

1 Lie on your back on the mat. Lift your legs off the floor until your knees are bent at a 90-degree angle, then cross your ankles. Your fingertips should rest on each side of your head, or you can rest your arms on each side of your body, with your palms flat on the floor.

cross your ankles

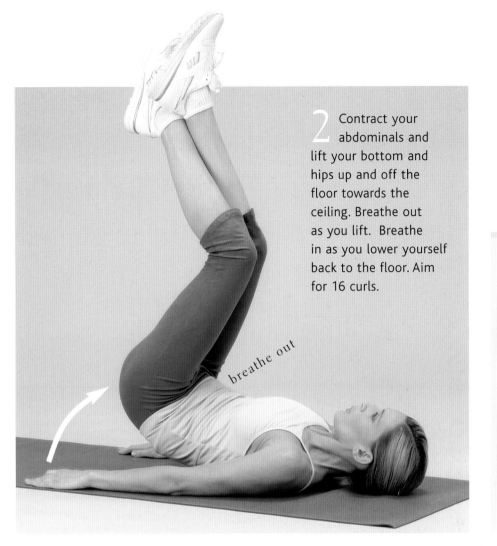

2 Contract your abdominals and lift your bottom and hips up and off the floor towards the ceiling. Breathe out as you lift. Breathe in as you lower yourself back to the floor. Aim for 16 curls.

breathe out

TRAINER TIPS

Try not to swing your legs back and forth to gain momentum; the movement should come from your core muscles.

Think of taking the movement up towards the ceiling.

REALLY WORK IT!

Once you can effectively curl upwards, move on to this version where you also lift your chest. This will give you a 'crunch' feeling. Lie on your back as before, with your knees bent, ankles crossed and fingertips on each side of your head.

Curl your legs and pelvis towards your ribcage, at the same time lifting your shoulders off the mat, curling them forwards towards your knees. Then lower yourself back to the floor. Aim for 16 curls.

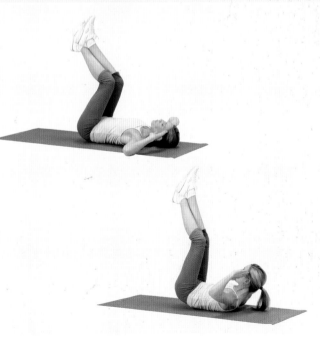

oblique CROSS-CRUNCH

This cross-crunch works the oblique
abdominal muscles that run along each
side of the torso. It helps with **tightening**
and defining the waist.

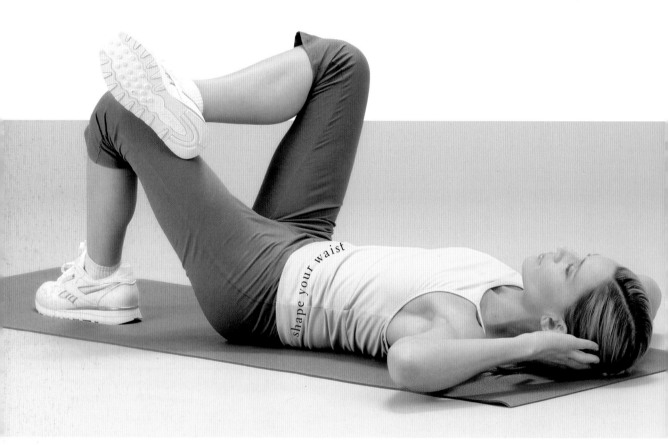

shape your waist

1 Lie on your back on the mat and place your
fingers on each side of your head. Cross your
right leg over your left knee. Breathe in and
contract your abdominals.

TRAINER TIP

Keep pushing your
bent knee back and
away from you.

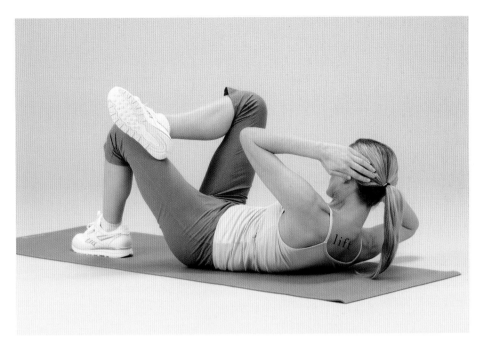

2 Breathe out as lift
your shoulders off
the mat and twist from
your waist to the right.
Your left elbow should
come across your chest
to your right knee.

3 Hold the twist at its maximum point for two
seconds, then return to your starting position.
Repeat on the other side. Aim for 16 cross-
crunches on each side.

side RAISE

This is **a great core exercise** that gives strength and tone. It is, however, a difficult exercise as it requires strength. Begin with the basic version where the knees are bent and one hand remains on the floor for stability.

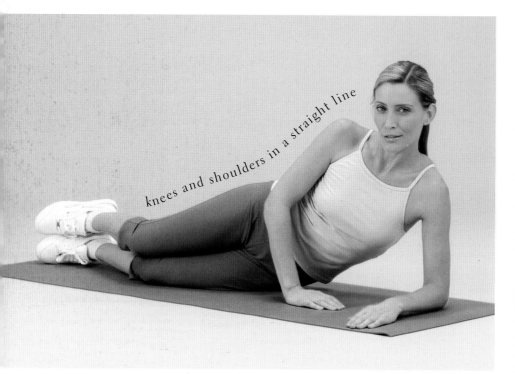

knees and shoulders in a straight line

TRAINER TIPS

Focus on a spot on the floor to help you concentrate.

Keep breathing throughout the exercise, but make sure you pull in your abdominal muscles the minute you start to lift off the floor.

Aim for perfect posture and alignment throughout.

1 Lie on your left side with your knees slightly bent. Your left elbow should be bent and under your shoulder and your right hand flat on the floor in front of your chest. Your shoulders and knees should be in a straight line.

2 Pull in your abdominals and lift your hips up until your body is in a straight line. Hold for five to ten seconds. Lower down gently, relax and repeat. Aim for ten lifts.

lift

REALLY WORK IT!

If you can hold the basic side raise for ten seconds, try the next level. Lie on your right side with your legs straight and your left foot resting on your right foot. Lift your hips upwards to raise yourself on both legs.

When you feel comfortable, take your left hand off the floor and place it on your left leg. Hold for ten seconds, then lower yourself back to the floor. Aim for ten lifts.

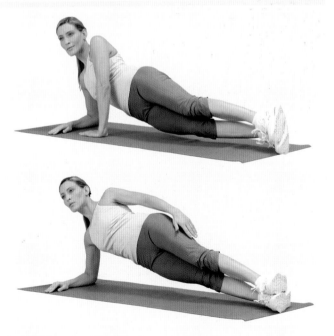

bicycle CRUNCH

The bicycle crunch is very effective on most of the **muscles throughout your mid-section**. It also helps to strengthen the lower stomach muscles, the rectus abdominus, the external and internus obliques and the hip flexors.

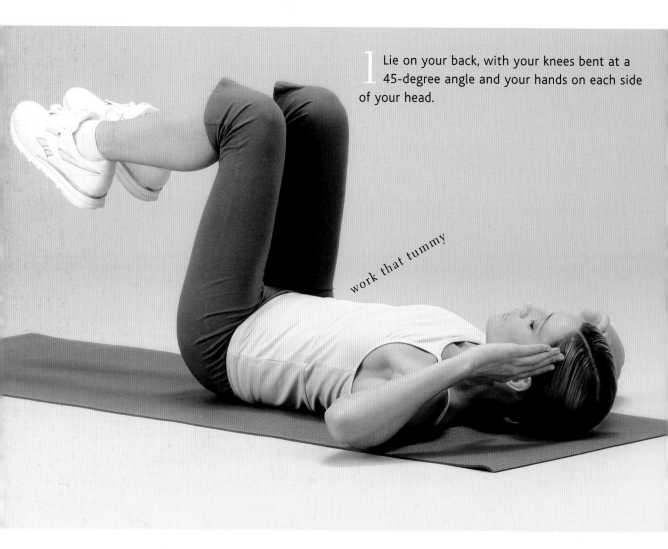

1 Lie on your back, with your knees bent at a 45-degree angle and your hands on each side of your head.

work that tummy

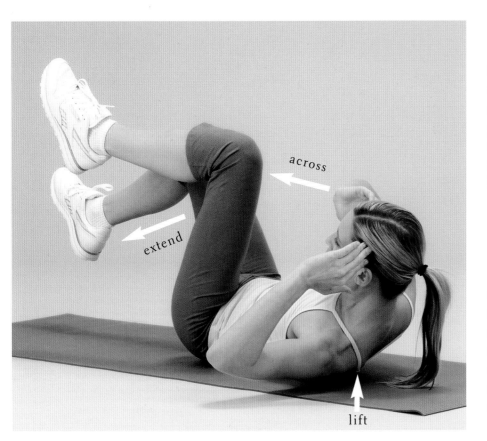

across

extend

lift

2 Lift your head and shoulders, and take your right elbow over to your left knee as you pull it towards your chest, at the same time extending your right leg straight out, keeping it off the floor.

3 Now change so that your left elbow goes across to your right knee and your left leg is extended out in front of you. The movement should look as if you are cycling. Aim for 16 crunches.

TRAINER TIPS

Focus on lifting your shoulders off the floor by contracting your abdominal muscles on each rotation.

Keep your shoulders and head off the floor throughout the exercise.

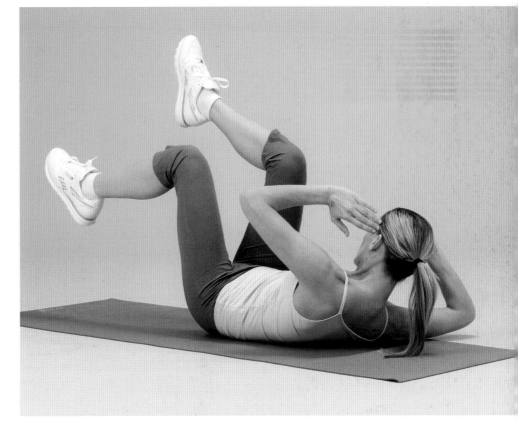

dumb-bell SIDE BEND

The aim of this exercise is to help work the waist and lengthen each side of the torso, improving posture and creating **a leaner, longer look**.

1 Stand straight, with your feet hip-width apart and your arms relaxed by your sides. Squeeze a hand weight in your right hand. Pull in your tummy and drop your shoulders, lengthening your spine.

TRAINER TIPS

Exhale as you stretch over to the side, keeping the hand weight away from the side of your body.

Ensure you keep your tummy muscles pulled in and your shoulders down.

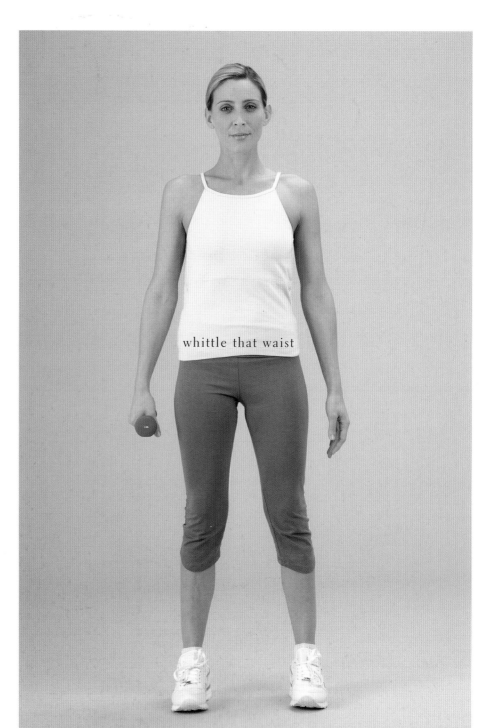

whittle that waist

2 Exhale as you stretch your left arm up and over your head, so that you bend to the right, stretching through the fingers of your left hand. At the same time let your right arm slide down your left side, keeping the hand weight slightly away from your body. Inhale as you come back up to the centre and your starting position. Repeat the exercise nine more times. Then change the weight over to your left hand. Aim for ten repetitions on each side.

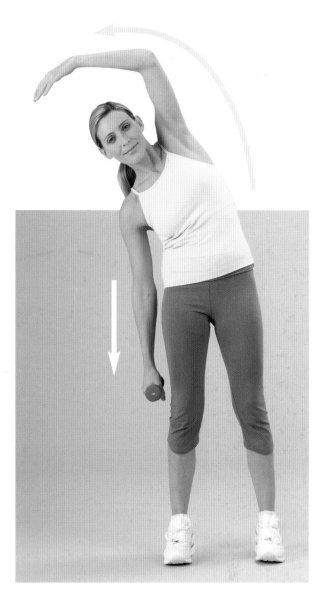

REALLY WORK IT!

Progress to holding a weight in each hand and extending them – with care – above the head and down the side of the body. Exhale as you stretch your right arm with the hand weight up and over your head, bending to the left. At the same time let your left arm slide down your left side, keeping the hand weight slightly away from your body. Inhale as you come back up to the centre. Aim for ten repetitions on each side.

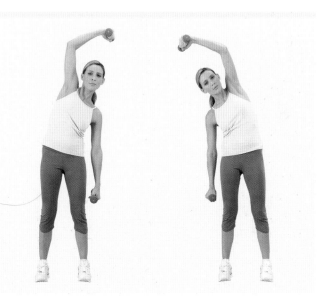

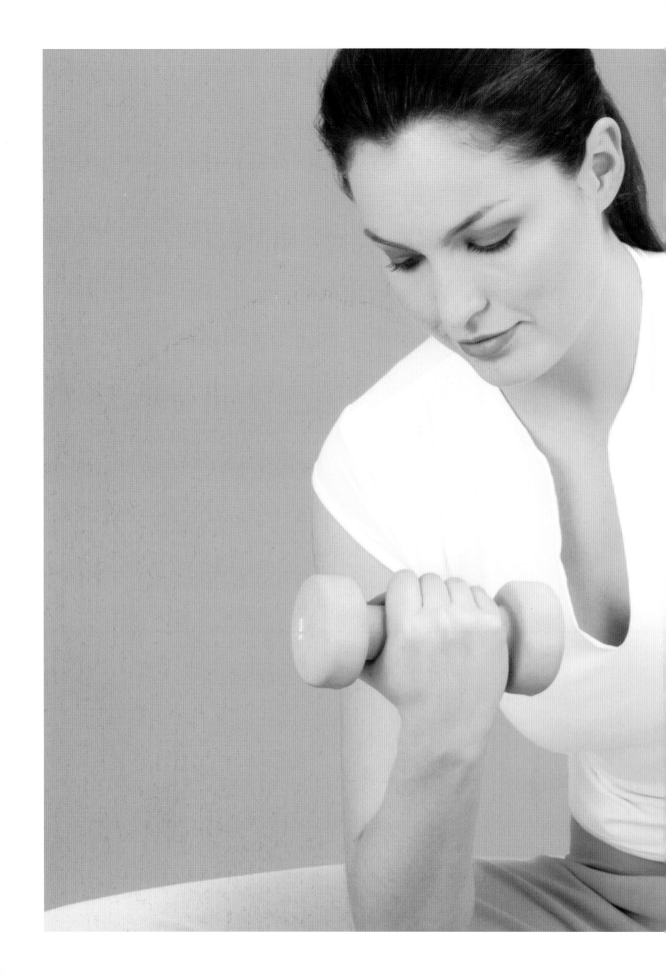

Arms and shoulders

triceps DIP

This exercise aims to tighten the muscle at the back of the arm, helping to **get rid of those bat wings**. You can do the triceps dip on a chair, bench or step, or even on the edge of the bed.

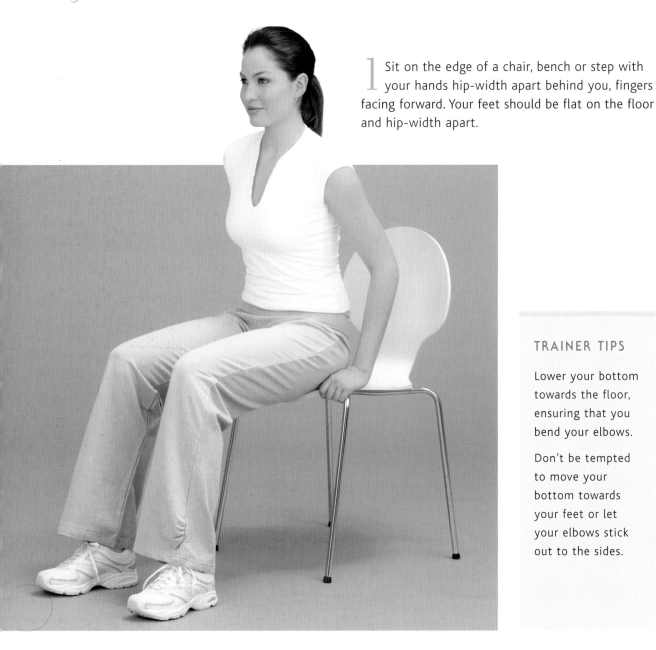

1 Sit on the edge of a chair, bench or step with your hands hip-width apart behind you, fingers facing forward. Your feet should be flat on the floor and hip-width apart.

TRAINER TIPS

Lower your bottom towards the floor, ensuring that you bend your elbows.

Don't be tempted to move your bottom towards your feet or let your elbows stick out to the sides.

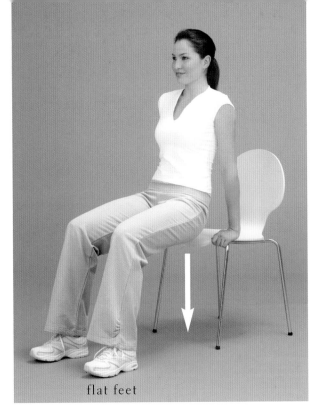

flat feet

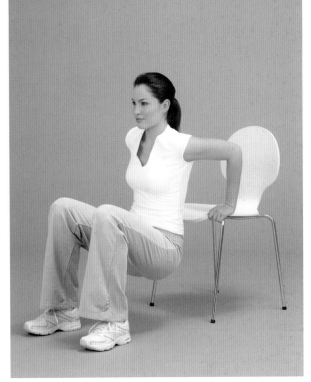

2 Pull in your tummy and, keeping your back straight, lift your body weight off the seat.

3 Lower your bottom towards the floor, bending your elbows. Make sure your elbows remain pointing backwards. Straighten your arms, push back up to the starting position and repeat, keeping your back close to the edge of the seat. Aim to do ten dips. Once you can achieve this, increase the number to 20.

REALLY WORK IT!

The further your feet are away from your body, the more the triceps muscle is worked. Sit on the edge of the chair, bench or step and extend your feet straight out in front of you, resting on your heels with your toes pointing towards the ceiling.

Lift your body weight off the seat and lower your bottom to the floor, bending your elbows and keeping your back straight. Straighten your arms and push back up, keeping your back close to the edge of the seat. Repeat 16 times.

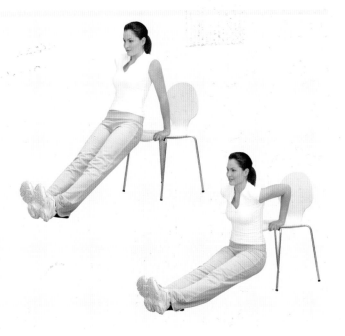

lateral dumb-bell RAISE

This dumb-bell raise helps to strengthen and tone the chest muscles (pectorals), which will **improve your bustline and your posture**.

TRAINER TIPS

Sitting on a chair or over the edge of a sofa may help to keep your back straight, giving you an enhanced technique – especially for those who have not used light hand weights before.

Keep your knees soft throughout the exercise and your back in a straight line.

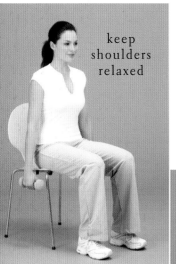

keep shoulders relaxed

1 Sit or stand with your feet hip-width apart. Hold a dumb-bell in each hand, resting them down by your sides or slightly in front of you.

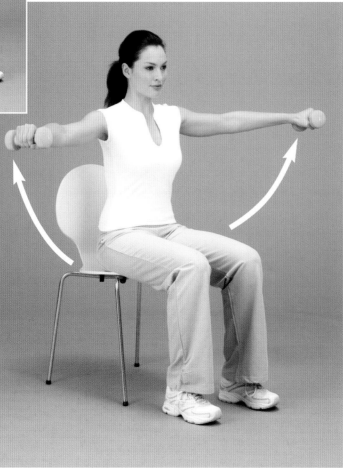

2 Inhale as you slowly lift your arms up to shoulder level in a controlled manner, squeezing your shoulder muscles as you do so. Hold for a second or two. Exhale as you lower back to the starting position. Aim for 16 lifts.

straight-arm PULL-OVER

The aim of this exercise is to **stretch the shoulder, arm and chest muscles,** whilst targeting the latissimi dorsi muscles as well as the lower body and core muscles.

1 Lie back with your shoulders on the ball, feet flat on the floor and hip-width apart. Hold a dumb-bell in each hand and extend your arms above your chest. Do not lock out your elbows and remember to keep your hips lifted.

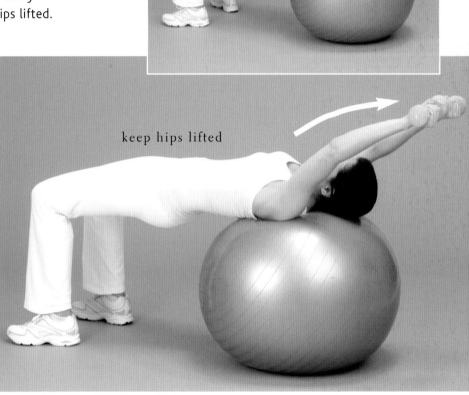

keep hips lifted

TRAINER TIPS

Keep your wrists straight and strong and your hips lifted throughout.

When you feel yourself getting tired through the mid-section, place the dumb-bells on the middle of your chest and lower your hips, until your buttocks touch the front of the ball and you can place the weights on the floor.

2 Breathe in as you lower the dumb-bells down behind your head. You will feel a stretch through your arms. Hold for a count of one, then breathe out as you bring the weight and your arms back to the starting position. Repeat. Aim for 16 pull-overs.

shoulder PRESS

The shoulder press can be done either sitting or standing. It strengthens the shoulder and **works the chest muscles.**

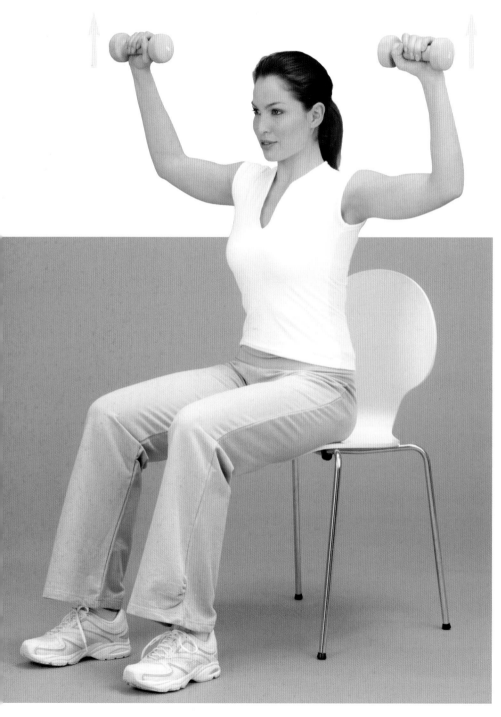

1 Sit or stand with your feet hip-width apart, holding a dumbbell in each hand. Lift the weights out to your sides, with your palms facing forward. Bend your elbows to a 90-degree angle.

TRAINER TIPS

Concentrate on squeezing the weights throughout the exercise.

Keep your chest lifted, but don't arch your back as you reach upwards.

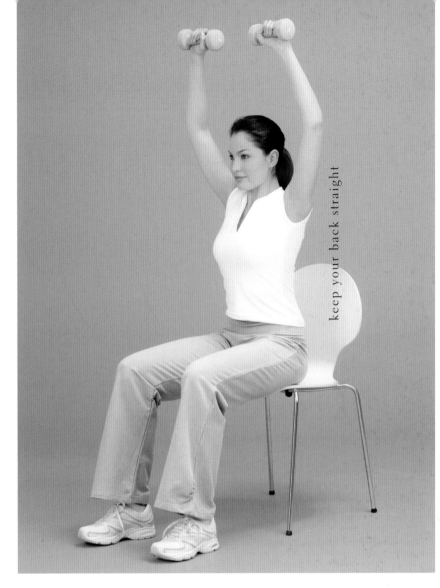

keep your back straight

2 Press the dumb-
bells up and
overhead until your
arms are extended.
Hold for a second, then
lower your arms back
down to your shoulders
in a controlled manner.
Do not let them drop
below the shoulder line.
Aim for 16 repetitions.

REALLY WORK IT!

To make this exercise more difficult, engage
your core muscles before you start. Sit on a
Swiss ball, with your feet hip-width apart. Keep
your arms bent, with your elbows at shoulder
level and bent to a 90-degree angle and your
palms facing outwards, holding the dumb-bells.
Tighten your abdominal muscles and press the
weights upwards, straightening your arms. Lower
your arms to the starting position and repeat.
Aim for 16 repetitions.

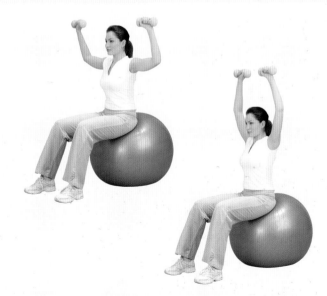

concentration biceps CURL

This exercise really works the biceps, making it an excellent exercise to shape and tone the front of your arms.

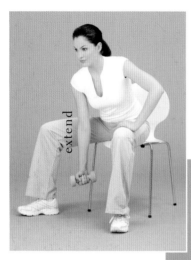

extend

1 Sit on the edge of a chair or bench with your legs apart. Hold the dumb-bell in your right hand, facing towards your right knee. Your left hand should rest on your left thigh, with fingers facing inwards. Extend your right arm fully until it is straight.

2 Curl the dumb-bell up towards your shoulder. Hold for a second and then, still squeezing the biceps, lower the dumb-bell with control. Repeat with the other hand. Aim for 16 curls.

TRAINER TIPS

Your biceps are usually stronger than your triceps, so you may find you can lift a heavier weight than normal. Or simply increase the number of repetitions you make.

Be careful not to use your chest when lifting.

biceps CURL

This variation of the biceps curl also helps to work the biceps muscle.

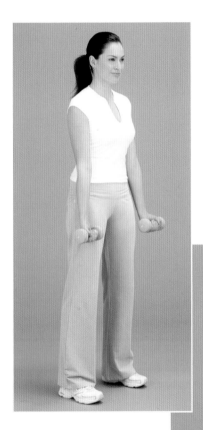

squeeze the weight

1 Stand or sit with your feet flat on the floor, hip-width apart, with a dumb-bell in each hand.

2 Keeping your elbows close to your sides, breathe out and bend them as you curl the dumb-bells towards your shoulders. Breathe in as you return the weight and your arms to the starting position. Aim for 16 curls.

TRAINER TIPS

Make sure you keep the movement controlled.

Do not allow the weight to swing down.

overhead triceps EXTENSION

This really works the triceps at the back of the arm, toning the muscle and helping to **get rid of those 'saddlebags'**. If you want to take the pressure off your back, do this exercise in a seated position. Perform this exercise slowly to get the best benefits.

1 Hold a dumb-bell in your left hand and lift it straight up over your head until it is perpendicular to the floor. Place your right hand around your left triceps for support.

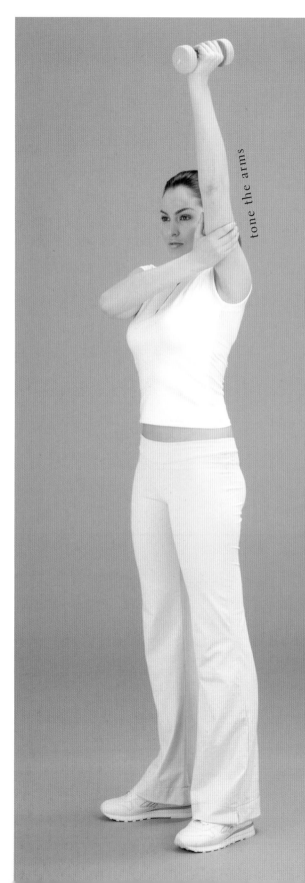

tone the arms

Make sure the
shoulders of
the working arm
are kept firm
throughout.

If you find this
exercise hard to
start with, use both
hands to hold the
weight until your
triceps strengthens.

2 Lower your left
arm back over
your shoulder and
behind your head,
bending the elbow
until the weight is
resting between
your shoulder blades.

3 With control, lift
the weight back
up above your head
towards the ceiling.
Repeat 16 times.

REALLY WORK IT!

For an advanced version of this exercise, lie
backwards on a Swiss ball, keeping it under your
shoulders and neck. Make sure your hips are
lifted and your feet are hip-width apart.

With a dumb-bell in each hand, lift your arms
up, with the palms facing towards you.

Bend your elbows at 90 degrees towards your
head. Slowly return your arms to the starting
position. Repeat 16 times.

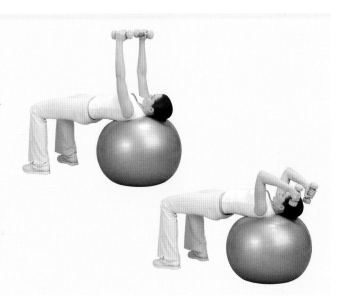

triceps KICKBACK

This is another very effective exercise to tone and **shape the upper arms**. You can do it using either one weight or two.

1 Stand with your feet hip-width apart and a dumb-bell in each hand. Bend over so that you are parallel to the floor, with your back straight and your abdominals pulled in and up.

2 Bend your elbows, then pull them up so that your knuckles are up to chest height.

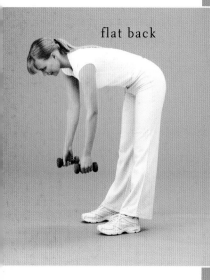

flat back

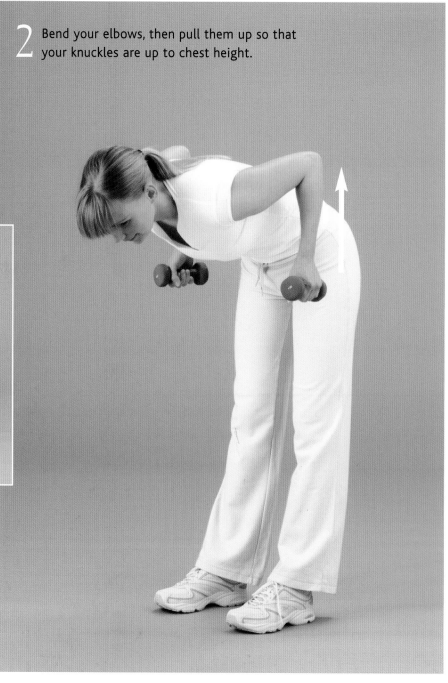

squeeze the muscles

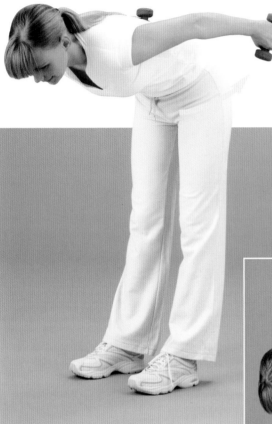

3 Extend your arms behind you, squeezing the triceps.

4 Lift your left leg straight out behind you, keeping a slight bend in the right knee. Return your leg and arms to the starting position. Repeat on the other side. Aim for 8–12 lifts.

TRAINER TIP

Keep your abdominal muscles pulled up towards your spine.

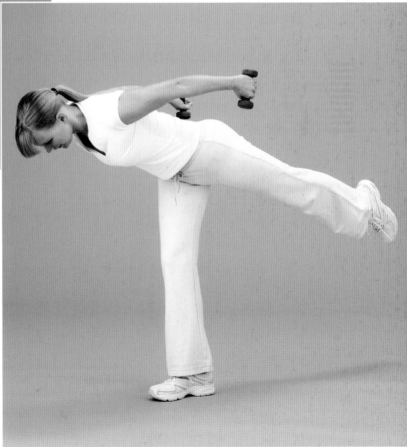

hammer CURL

The hammer curl works the biceps muscle, helping to **tone the upper arms**.

1 Hold a dumb-bell in each hand down by your sides, with the palms facing towards your body. Stand with your feet hip-width apart.

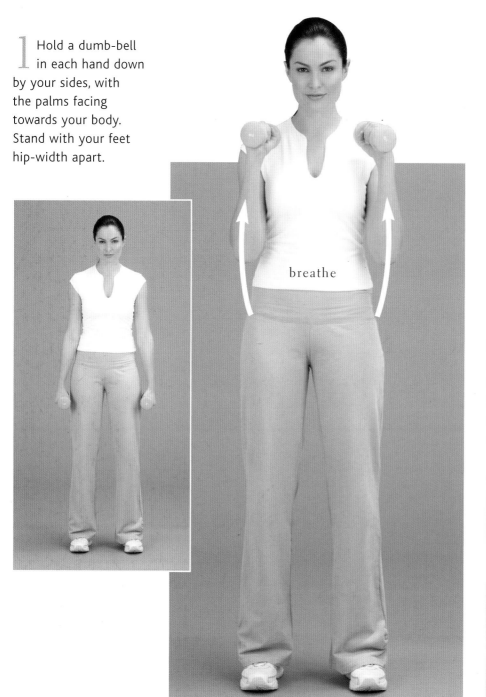

breathe

2 Raise your arms to your shoulders, bending your elbows and keeping them close to your sides. Bring them back to the starting position and repeat. Aim for 16 curls.

TRAINER TIP

Make sure your thumbs are pointing towards you and that your shoulders are relaxed and down.

reverse FLY

This exercise works the posterior deltoid muscle, at the top of the back of the arm. It shapes the shoulders and upper back.

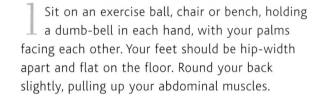

1 Sit on an exercise ball, chair or bench, holding a dumb-bell in each hand, with your palms facing each other. Your feet should be hip-width apart and flat on the floor. Round your back slightly, pulling up your abdominal muscles.

2 Keeping a slight bend in your elbows, raise your arms and dumb-bells up and out to the sides until they are parallel to the floor. Slowly lower your arms back to the starting position. Aim for 16 lifts.

keep shoulders down

TRAINER TIPS

Keep the abdominals pulled up throughout the exercise.

Squeeze your shoulder blades together as you lift the weight, but do not raise your shoulders.

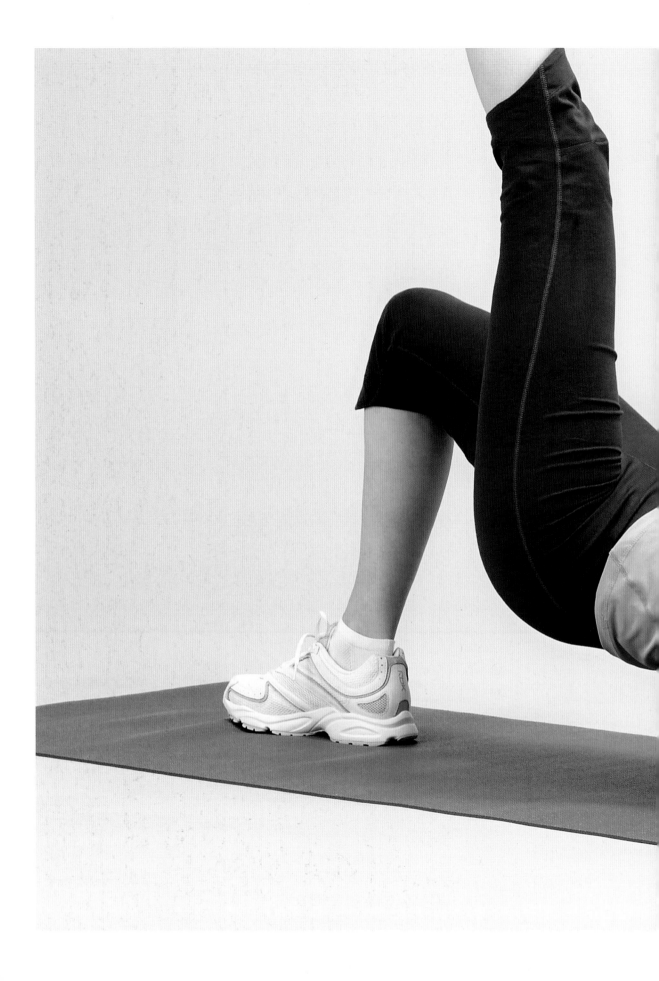

Beautifying
the bottom

SQUAT with dumb-bell

This exercise is guaranteed to help **tone and lift the bottom**. It is great for really working the gluteal muscles and the thighs.

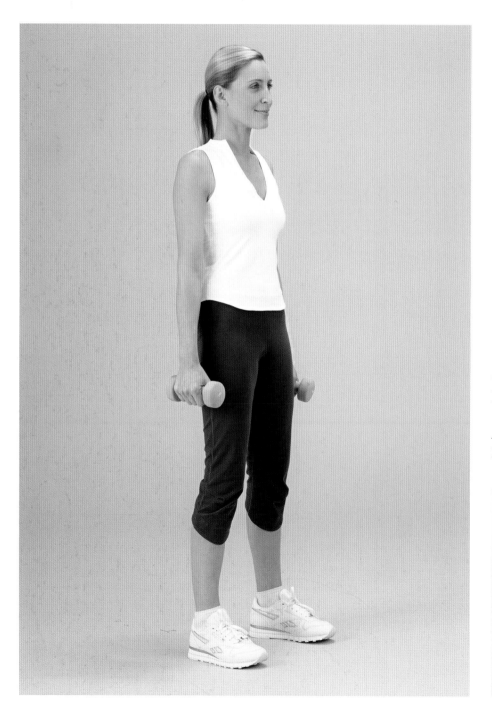

1 Stand with your feet hip-width apart, arms down by your sides and a dumb-bell in each hand, held just on the outside of your thighs.

TRAINER TIP

Breathe out as you squat down and breathe in as you return to the starting position.

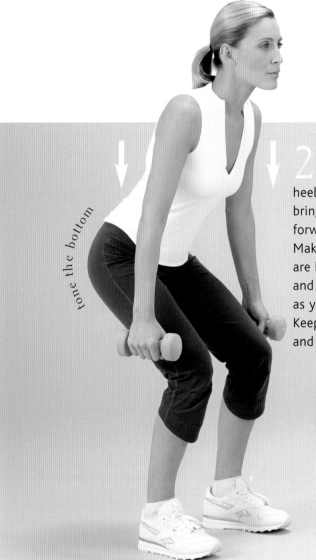

tone the bottom

2 Keeping the weight in your heels, bend your knees, bringing your shoulders forward over the knees. Make sure your knees are behind your toes and contract your abs as you squat down. Keep your back straight and look ahead.

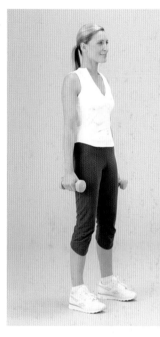

3 Contract the glutes (bottom) and hamstrings as you return to the starting position and repeat. Aim for 16 squats.

REALLY WORK IT!

To make the exercise more challenging, lift the dumb-bells to shoulder level as you squat. Stand as before, then bend your knees, bringing your shoulders forward over them, and at the same time raise your arms out to shoulder level. Lower your arms back down and return to the starting position. Repeat. Aim for 16 squats.

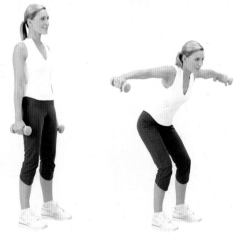

bridge-bottom LIFT

This lift helps to strengthen the quadriceps, thighs and gluteus maximus and minimus muscles of the buttocks, which will tone your bottom, making it **tighter and more lifted**. It works the abdominal muscles and lower back, too.

TRAINER TIPS

Pull up the pelvic-floor muscles as you tilt your pelvis up.

Do not use your lower back to lift your buttocks. There should be no strain through your lower back.

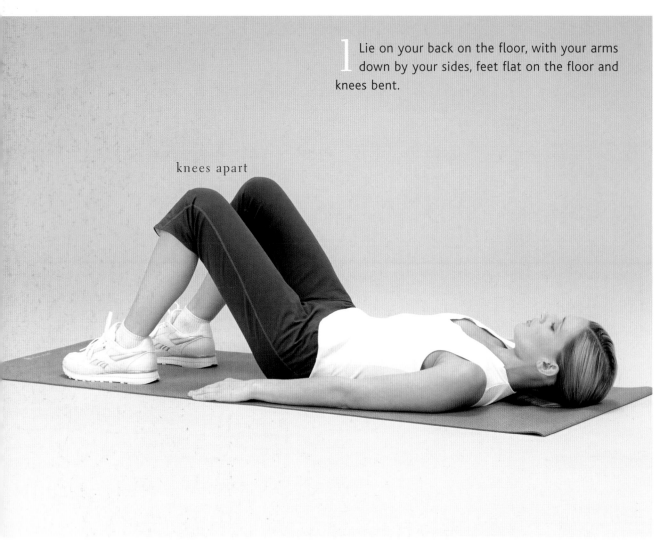

1 Lie on your back on the floor, with your arms down by your sides, feet flat on the floor and knees bent.

knees apart

2 Lift your bottom off the mat, keeping your feet and knees apart. As you begin to lift, contract your abdominal muscles, drawing your belly button down to your spine. Your hips and knees should now be in a straight line. Squeeze your bottom on each lift. Lower yourself slowly down and repeat. Aim for 16 lifts.

REALLY WORK IT!

Using the edge of a step or chair makes the lift higher and works the gluteal muscles harder. Lie on your back on the floor as before. Place your heels on the edge of a step or chair, keeping your knees bent.

Lift your bottom off the floor by squeezing it until your body is in a straight line with your hips, knees and chest. Lower your hips slightly, then lift again, using your bottom.
Aim for 20 lifts.

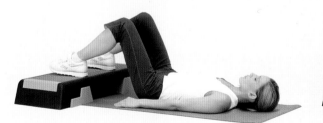

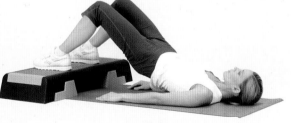

donkey KICK

The aim of this exercise is to target your gluteal muscles. It is also great at helping to sculpt and tone your bottom.

1 Kneel on your elbows and knees, keeping your knees hip-width apart and clasping your hands together. Pull in your abdominal muscles and breathe out.

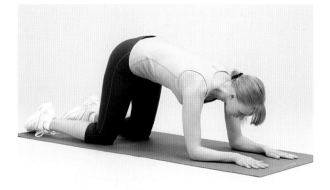

flat foot

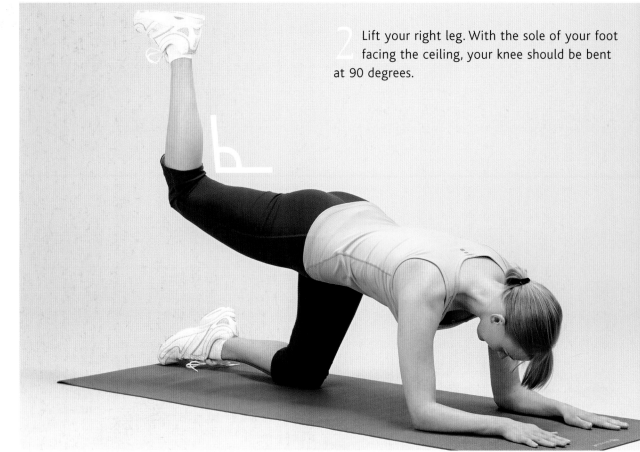

2 Lift your right leg. With the sole of your foot facing the ceiling, your knee should be bent at 90 degrees.

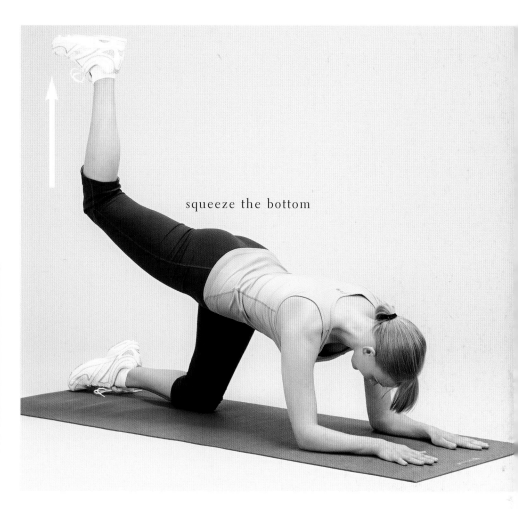

squeeze the bottom

Keep your abdominal muscles tight, pulling up your pelvic-floor muscles (the ones that you use to stop your urine flow) throughout the exercise. It is your bottom muscles that do the work, not the leg.

3 Push the right leg up, squeezing your bottom, and then back down towards the ground – but not touching the floor. Repeat nine more times on the right leg. Lower the leg and repeat on the left leg. Aim for ten lifts to begin with; as you improve aim for 20 lifts on each leg.

REALLY WORK IT!

Perform the exercise exactly as before, but this time use ankle weights to increase the intensity. Aim for three repetitions of 16 lifts on each leg.

standing PUSH-BACK

Another amazing exercise for the bottom, this will help to lift and tone the bottom while **working the hamstrings and quadriceps.**

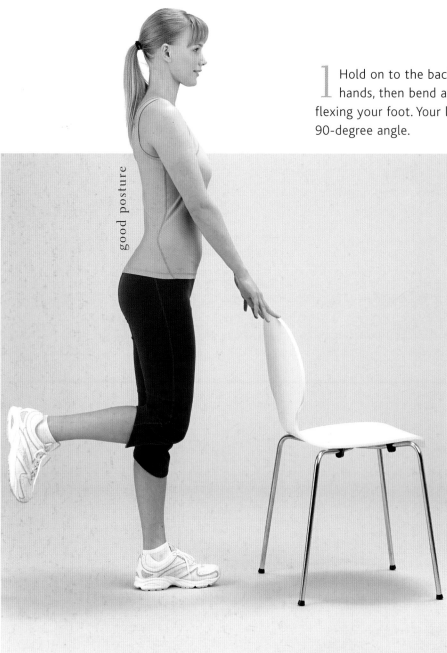

good posture

1 Hold on to the back of a chair with both hands, then bend and lift your right knee, flexing your foot. Your leg should be at a 90-degree angle.

TRAINER TIPS

Keep the abdominal muscles pulled in throughout the whole of this exercise.

Also check your posture: your back should be straight and your shoulders must be pulled down and back.

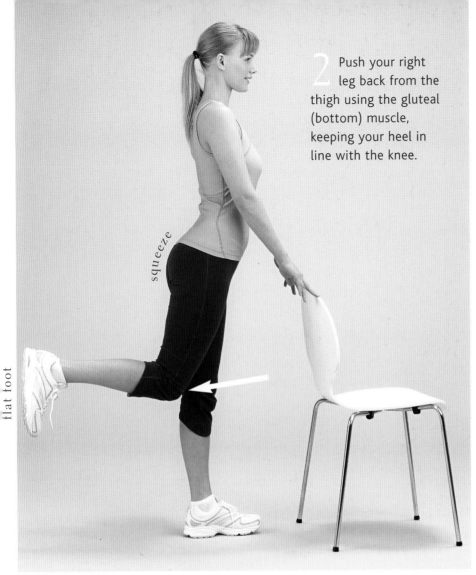

squeeze

flat foot

2 Push your right leg back from the thigh using the gluteal (bottom) muscle, keeping your heel in line with the knee.

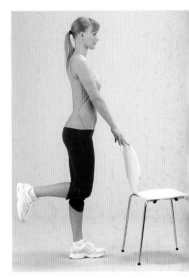

3 Bring your knee back to the starting position. Aim for 16 push-backs on each leg.

REALLY WORK IT!

Perform the same exercise as before, but this time use a wrap-around ankle weight to increase its intensity and give an added stretch. Aim for 16 push-backs on each leg.

cross-over SQUAT

More intense than an ordinary squat,
this exercise works the bottom and thighs,
as well as the quadriceps muscles and the
abdominal muscles.

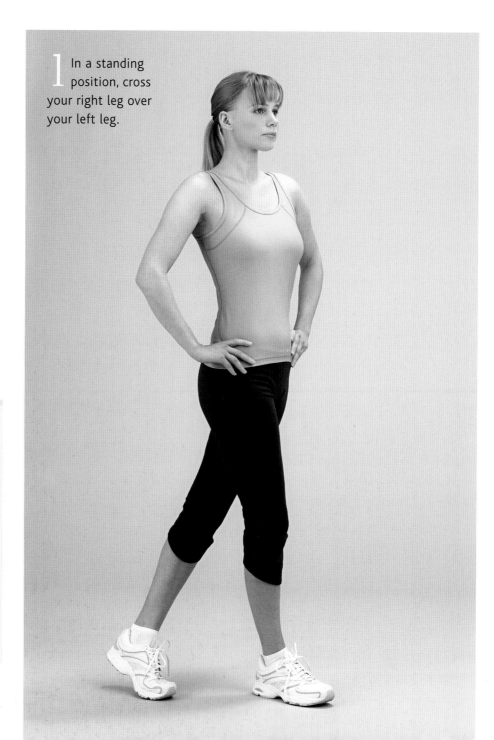

1 In a standing position, cross your right leg over your left leg.

TRAINER TIP

This requires you to have good balance. So perform it slowly, making sure that you maintain a good posture throughout.

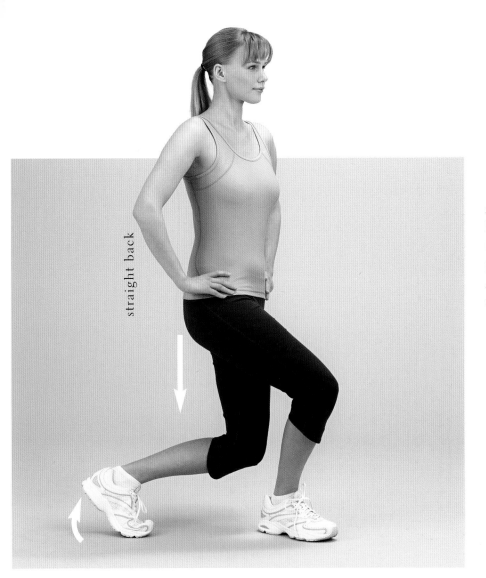

straight back

2 Place your hands on your hips and squat down, lifting the heel of the left leg. Return to the starting position and repeat. Aim for 16 squats on each leg.

REALLY WORK IT!

In this version you squat while holding a dumb-bell in each hand. Cross your right leg over your left leg, as before.

Holding a dumb-bell in each hand, cross your arms over your chest with your palms facing outwards. Now squat down, lifting the heel of the left leg. Return to the starting position and repeat. Aim for 16 squats on each leg.

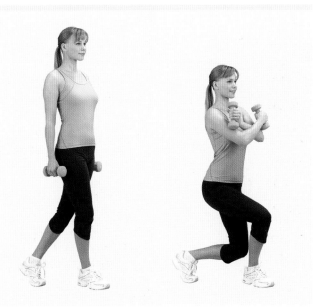

swimming KICK

The swimming kick works on the quadriceps and gluteals and is quite difficult to do. However, if you persist, you will find that it gives great shape and tone to your bottom and **makes your thighs much stronger**.

pert bottom

1 Lie face down on the floor on the mat. Place your arms under your head. Your legs should be together and your thighs turned inward, by rolling your feet out and pointing your toes.

TRAINER TIP

Keep your back relaxed, but pull up your abdominals before you commence the exercise and during the lifts.

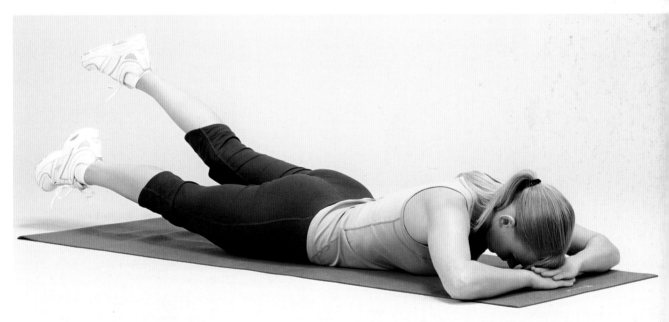

2 Pull up your abdominal muscles and lift your legs, including the front of your thighs, off the floor.

3 With your legs elevated off the floor, keep your legs straight and your body flat on the ground. Kick your legs up and down slowly as if you were swimming. Aim for 20 kicks.

one-legged HIP RAISE

This hip raise not only tones your bottom and stretches the gluteal muscles, but also **works on your hamstrings and lower back**.

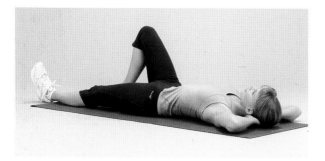

1 Lie on your back on the mat and bend one knee, keeping the other leg stretched straight out on the floor.

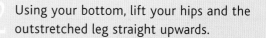

lengthen the hamstring

2 Using your bottom, lift your hips and the outstretched leg straight upwards.

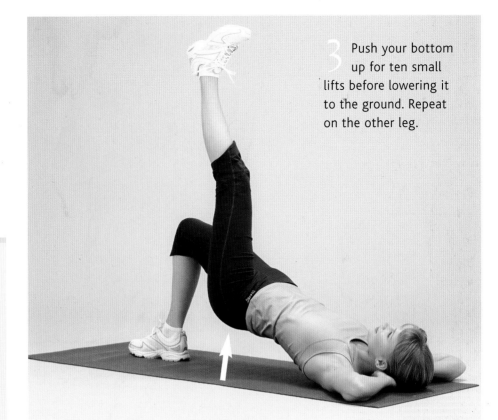

3 Push your bottom up for ten small lifts before lowering it to the ground. Repeat on the other leg.

TRAINER TIP

Make sure you are using the bottom to lift upwards, not your lower back.

REALLY WORK IT!

To make this exercise harder, lie on the floor with your feet on a Swiss ball and your knees straight.

Press your feet into the ball and lift your hips off the floor, with your arms on the floor on each side of you.

Lift your right leg off the ball, bending your knee towards your chest. Then lift your bottom and right leg up, keeping the ball still. Do ten small pushes towards the ceiling, using your bottom. Lower your leg and repeat on the other side.

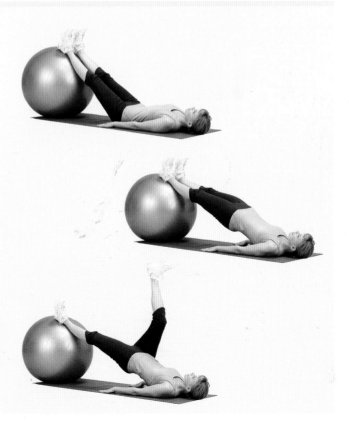

knee JACKS

This works the adductor and abductor muscles of the thigh, as well as your bottom.

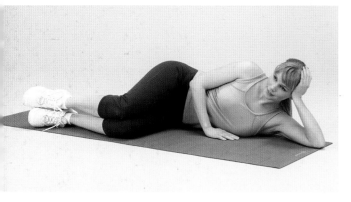

1 Lie on your left side, with the knees bent at 90 degrees to the body. Rest on your left elbow with your right hand flat on the mat in front of you.

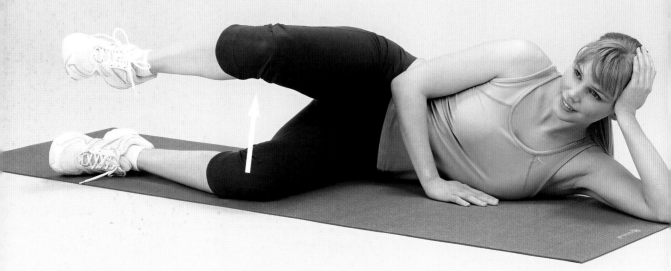

2 Lift your right knee up, keeping the ankle in line with the knee.

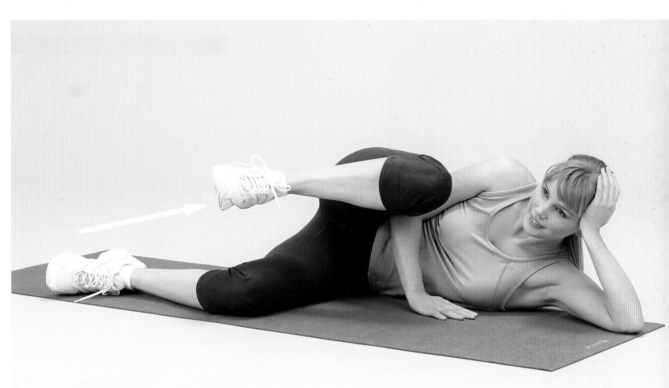

TRAINER TIP

Always keep
the movements
controlled and
squeeze the inner
thigh muscle.

3 Bring the right knee in towards your chest
and then push the leg straight back out,
straightening the knee and the thigh. Pull the
knee back in towards the chest. Make sure you
do not lean backwards as you lift your leg. Aim
for 16 jacks on each side.

REALLY WORK IT!

Add an ankle weight to increase the intensity
and strengthen the thigh. Keep your working leg
straight and in line with your hips.

Lift the right knee to a 90 degree angle. Pull the
knee towards the chest and then extend the leg
straight out. Aim for 10 jacks on each side.

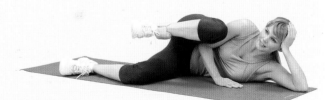

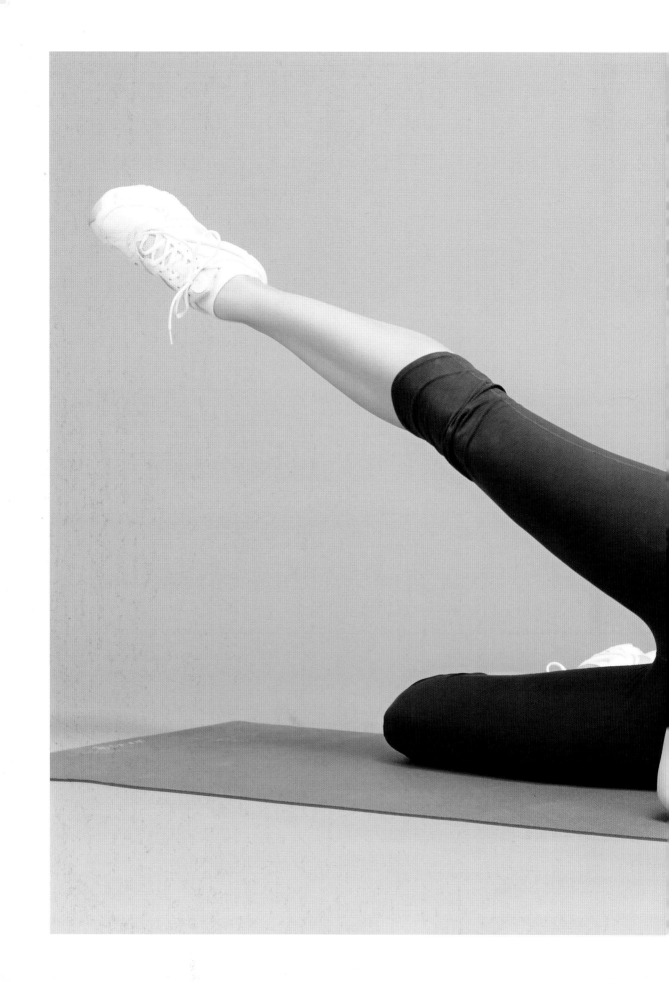

Perfect pins

leg LUNGE

This is one of the best leg exercises to build strength and **give shape to the legs**. Lunges help to tone the thighs, quadriceps and hamstrings. They are very versatile – you can perform them forwards, backwards, sideways or walking, to increase their intensity.

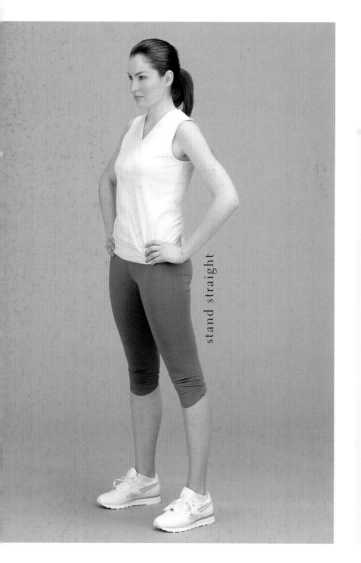

stand straight

1 Stand with your feet about 1 m (3 ft) apart and your hands on your hips.

TRAINER TIPS

Be aware of your posture: stand with your back straight and your shoulders drawn back and down. Pull in your abdominals before you begin and keep them tight.

If you feel unstable, hold on to the back of a chair for support until you have greater control.

2 Take a large step forward with your right leg, bending your left knee and lowering it towards the floor. At the same time lift your left heel off the floor. Your left knee should be pointing straight ahead and your right knee should be directly over your right foot. At first you may find that you do not lunge very far, but this will improve as you get stronger and fitter. Keep your shoulders in line with your hips, so that you don't tip forward.

step forward

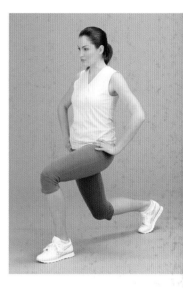

3 Then, using your bottom and thigh, push back up to the starting position. Repeat on the other side. Aim for 16 lunges on each leg.

REALLY WORK IT!

To make this exercise more challenging, you can use dumb-bells. Simply place a dumb-bell in each hand and hold them down by your sides as you lunge. Aim for 16 lunges on each leg.

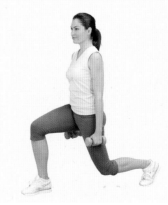

one-legged SQUAT

The one-legged squat targets your legs and buttocks, but adds another dimension as it **challenges your balance**, too. Good posture is needed at all times to make this exercise as effective as possible.

TRAINER TIP

Try looking in the mirror to keep your back straight and ensure that your abdominals are pulled in throughout the exercise.

1 Stand on both feet, then bend your right knee so that your right foot touches the side of your left knee. Point your toes downwards. Hold your arms out to the sides at shoulder height.

2 Extend your right foot forward, pointing the toes. Bend your left knee, lowering your body as far as you can, but not beyond 90 degrees. Hold for a count of four, then repeat. Aim for 12 squats. Keeping your body upright, slowly straighten your left knee and return to the starting position. Repeat on the left leg.

keep shoulders down

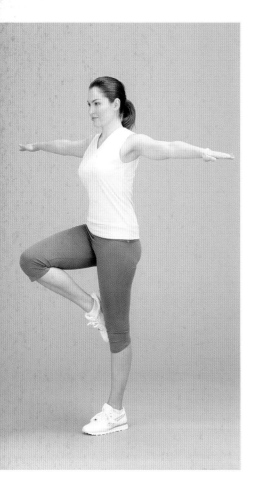

standing side LIFT

This standing lift helps to strengthen the buttocks, hamstrings and inner thigh muscles, the adductors.

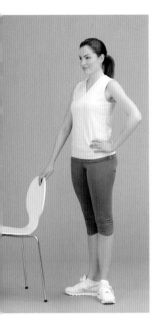

1 Hold on to the back of a chair for support. Stand with your left hand on your left hip. Place your heels together, with your feet turned out at a 45-degree angle. Make sure your legs are straight. Tighten your buttocks and pull in your abdominals.

2 Lift your left leg out to the side, keeping the foot flexed. Lift only as high as you comfortably can without letting your waist or hips rotate. Lower back to the standing leg, but do not put the left foot back on the ground as you lift again. Aim for 16 lifts on each side.

pull in

TRAINER TIPS

Make sure your hips face forward as you lift your leg, turning your raised thigh outwards.

Keep your back straight and your abdominals pulled in.

REALLY WORK IT!

To make this exercise more difficult, perform it as before, but add a wrap-around ankle weight to your working leg to increase the intensity of the lift. Aim for 16 lifts on each side.

inner thigh LIFT

Continuing to work on the inner thighs, this exercise will really help to **strengthen the adductor muscles**.

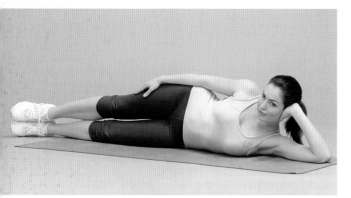

1 Lie on your left side on the mat, with your left elbow bent and supporting your head. Your legs should be in a straight line from your body, with your right hand resting on your right hip.

TRAINER TIP

Make sure your body is in a straight line as you lift and that your hips do not roll inwards.

2 Bend the right knee and place the right foot over the left leg and flat on the mat.

push hips forward

3 Breathe out as you lift your left leg, keeping the thigh off the mat and the leg straight. The toes should be flexed. Breathe in as you release the leg down. Make sure it does not touch the floor, and lift it again. Aim for 16 lifts on each leg.

foot flat

REALLY WORK IT!

To make this exercise harder, perform it as before, but add a wrap-around ankle weight to the leg that you are lifting. Aim for 16 lifts on each leg.

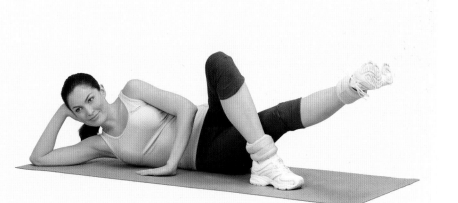

double leg LIFT

This exercise **works the thighs and the abdominals.** When you lift the legs together, you also work the buttocks and inner thighs.

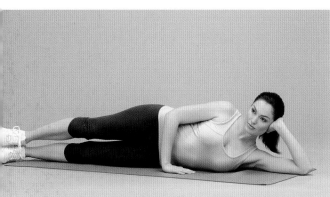

1 Lie on your left side on the mat, with your right leg on top of the left. Your left elbow should be bent and your hand supporting your head; your right hand should be flat on the floor in front of you. Lift your ribcage slightly from the mat. Check your body is in a straight line from your shoulders to your ankles.

keep legs straight

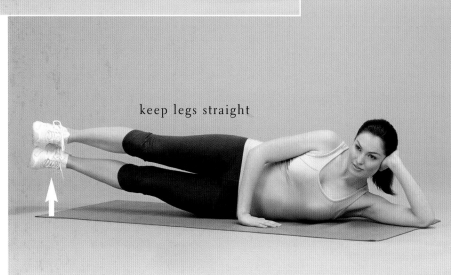

TRAINER TIPS

Do not push on your hand to help you to lift your legs.

Keep your abdominals tight throughout the exercise.

2 Breathe out and lift both legs from the mat, keeping them straight and the inner thighs together. Breathe in and slowly lower your legs back down, but make sure they do not touch the floor. Aim for ten lifts on each side.

single leg LIFT

This leg lift strengthens the gluteal muscles, the hips and buttocks and the hip-flexor muscles. You may find that your legs ache to begin with, but this will ease.

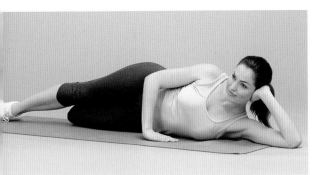

1 Lie on your left side in a straight line, with your left elbow bent and your left hand supporting your head. Place your right hand in front of you for support.

2 Bend your left knee underneath you and lift the right leg as high as you can, breathing out as you lift. Keeping the leg as straight as possible, hold for a count of two. Lower the leg back down, but do not let it touch the ground. Lift again. Aim for 16 lifts on each leg.

TRAINER TIP

Check that you are lying with your shoulders and hips in a straight line.

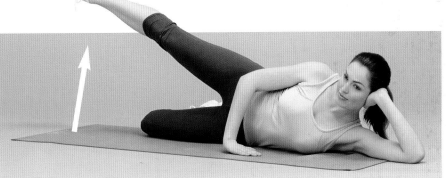

REALLY WORK IT!

Once you feel comfortable with the leg lift, add an ankle weight to the leg you are lifting. Start with a light weight and build up. Perform the exercise as before, and make sure your hips do not roll back and that your weight is kept pressed forward. Aim for 16 lifts on each leg.

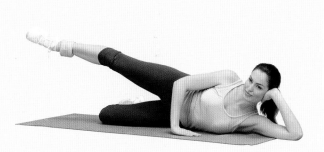

calf RAISE

To tone and shape the lower part of your legs – your calves – this exercise is a 'must'.

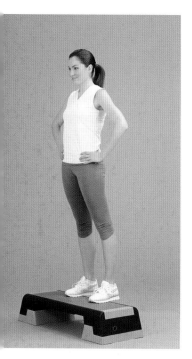

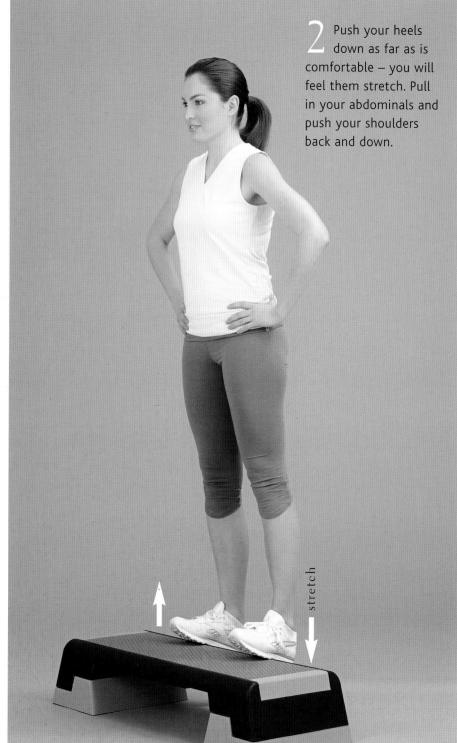

2 Push your heels down as far as is comfortable – you will feel them stretch. Pull in your abdominals and push your shoulders back and down.

stretch

1 Stand with the balls of your feet on a step. Your feet should be slightly apart and your toes pointing forwards. Place your hands on your hips, or hold on to something if you feel unbalanced.

TRAINER TIPS

Keep the knee pulled up, but not locked, during this exercise.

Bending and straightening the knees during this raise will take the tension out of your calves.

pull up the thighs

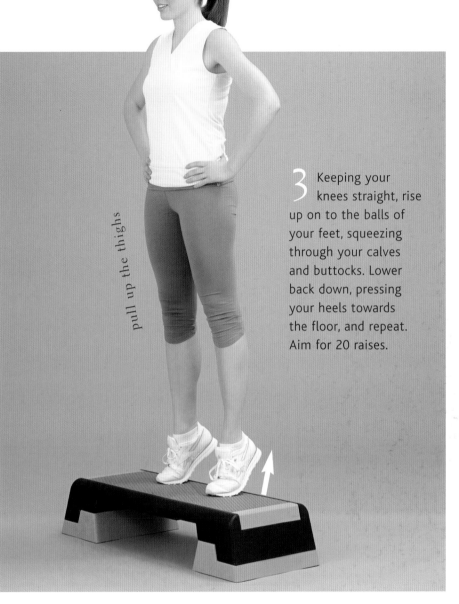

3 Keeping your knees straight, rise up on to the balls of your feet, squeezing through your calves and buttocks. Lower back down, pressing your heels towards the floor, and repeat. Aim for 20 raises.

REALLY WORK IT!

To increase the intensity of the exercise, perform it as before, but rise up on your left foot, crossing your right foot behind your left heel. Aim for 20 raises and then change feet.

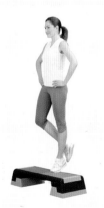

dancer's PLIÉ

A classic dancer's exercise, this helps to tone and **strengthen your lower body**. It works the legs, hips, bottom, hamstrings and calves, too.

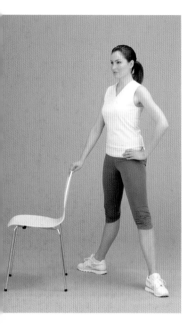

1 Hold on to the back of a chair with your right hand and stand with your feet wide apart, facing outwards, and your left hand on your hip. Breathe out and pull in your abdominals, keeping your back straight and your shoulders pressed down and back.

2 Bend both knees, keeping your knees over your toes. As you push down, make sure your knees do not roll inwards and that your feet stay flat on the floor. Hold for a count of two and then, breathing in slowly, return to the starting position. Aim for 16 pliés.

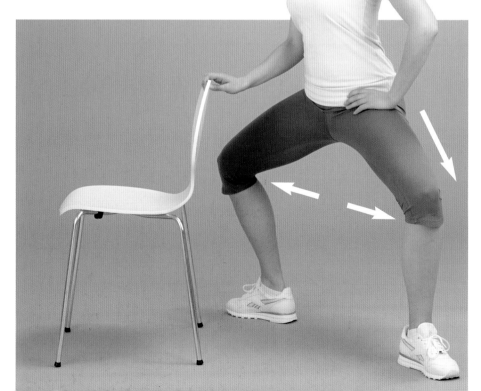

dancer's ARABESQUE

The arabesque works the quadriceps, thighs and all the bottom muscles, the gluteals. In addition **the hip flexors are targeted**, along with your back.

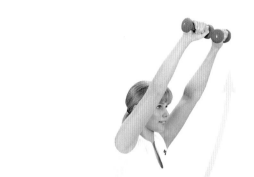

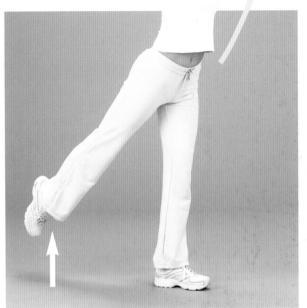

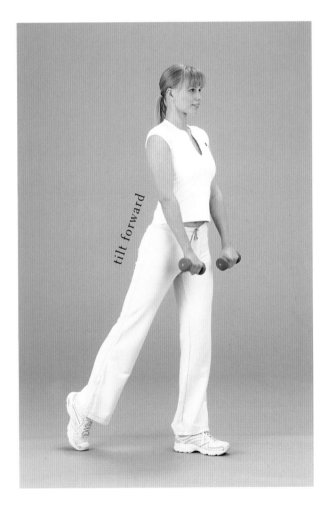

tilt forward

1 Stand with your right leg stretched behind you. Hold a weight in each hand at your sides. Slightly incline your body forward from the hips, keeping the back straight and your head up.

TRAINER TIPS

Keep your back straight and your hips facing forward to protect your back.

Leave the weights and hold on to the back of a chair if you need some support.

2 Breathe out as you lift your right leg as high as you comfortably can. At the same time lift both weights out in front of you and up to your head, keeping them in front of your shoulders. Hold for a count of two. Lower the leg and arms down and repeat on the left leg. Aim for 16 lifts.

side TURNERS

This exercise with help to tone your inner thigh and works on your hip flexors.

1 Lie on your left side with your left elbow bent and your left hand supporting your head. Bend both knees at a 90 degree angle so that the right knee and leg is resting on the left one.

TRAINER TIP

Make sure the foot of the working leg is always lower than the knee when you lift the leg.

2 Lift the left knee up, keeping the ankle lower than the knee.

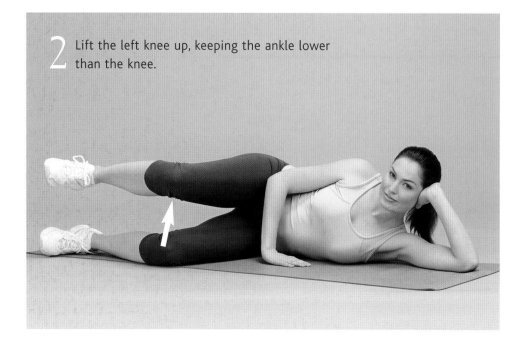

3 Continue lifting the right knee and then turn it out to the side, using the rotation in the hip and bottom. Bring the knee back in but do not let it come all the way back to the starting position before you rotate it back again. Aim to do 16 turns.

TRAINER TIP

Make sure your abdominals are pulled in before you begin, and that you draw up your pelvic-floor muscles.

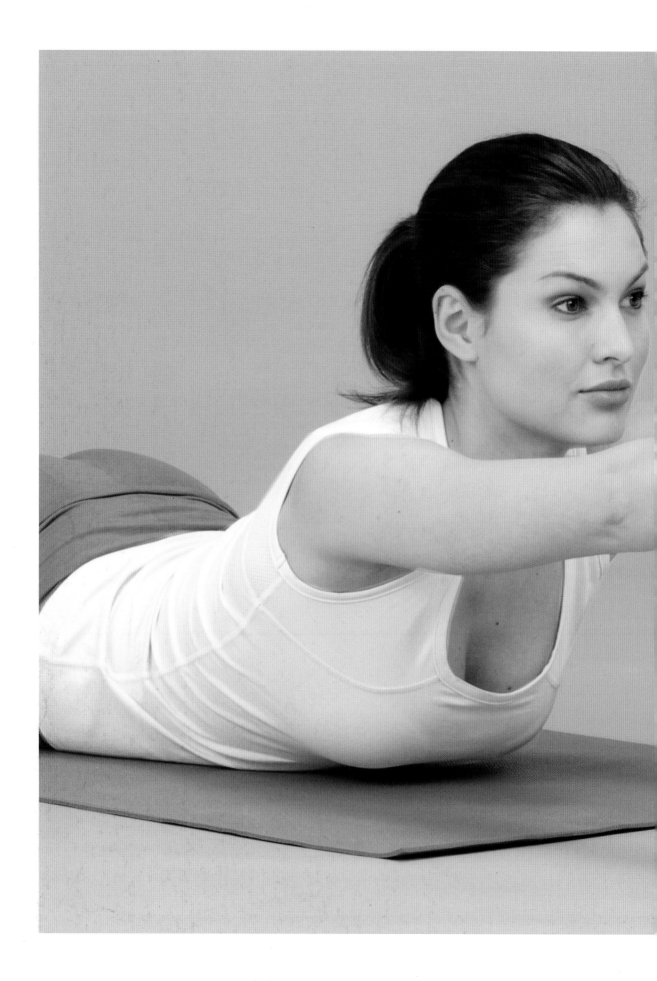

Chest and back

dumb-bell FLY

This exercise works the chest muscles to tone the chest area.

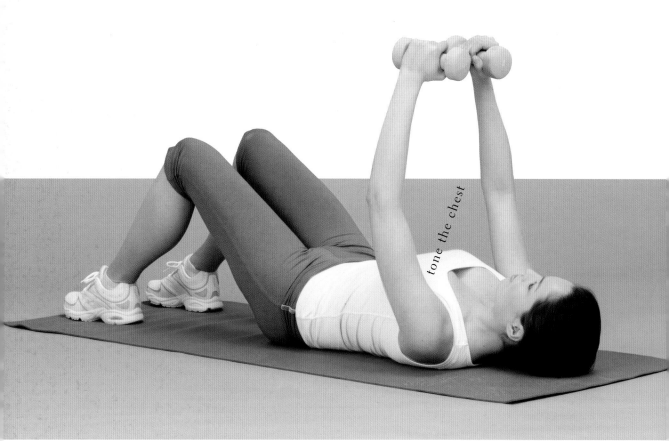

tone the chest

1 Lie on the mat with your feet flat on the floor and your knees bent. Hold a dumb-bell in each hand above your chest; your knuckles should be facing each other.

TRAINER TIP

If you contract your chest muscles at the top of the movement, you will get the full toning benefits.

2 Keeping a natural arch in your back, open your arms as if tracing a large arc outwards, until your elbows are down to the levels of your shoulders. Slowly push back up to the starting position. Aim for 16 repetitions.

REALLY WORK IT!

Use a Swiss ball to perform the same exercise, but concentrate on keeping it still and maintaining the correct posture by keeping your hips lifted. Lying on your back with your shoulders against the ball, keep the ball steady. Take your weights out to shoulder level on each side, keeping a soft bend in the elbow.

Bring the weights in above your head and over your chest in a large arc. Aim for 16 repetitions.

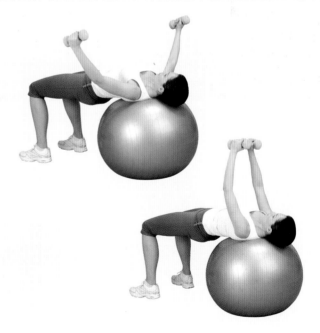

chest SQUEEZE

Using your own resistance will help the muscles around the chest to tone, and standing straight with good posture will make the upper body appear taller and more defined.

TRAINER TIP

Concentrate on pushing your hands together and squeezing your arm muscles.

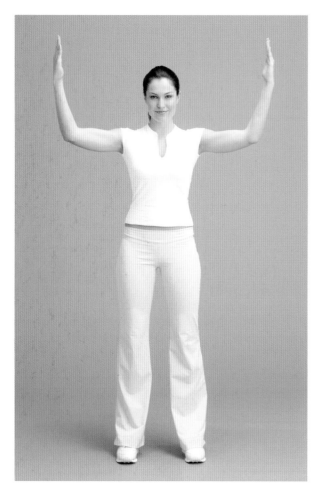

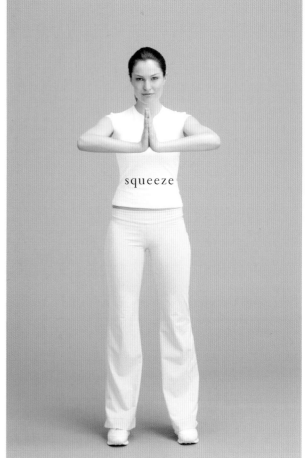

squeeze

1 Stand straight with your feet hip-width apart and your arms bent at the elbows and level with the shoulders. Your palms should face inwards. Relax your shoulders down and pull in your abdominals.

2 Bring the palms of your hands in together across the chest and squeeze them against each other. Your elbows should be raised to shoulder level and should go out to the sides. Squeeze hard for a count of one, relax and squeeze. Aim for 20 squeezes.

upright ROW

The upright row works the trapezius muscle, which runs from the neck to the shoulders and down the back. It also **tones the front of the shoulders** and gives shape to the upper body.

TRAINER TIP

As you lift, try not to raise your shoulders, keep them pressed down and your back long, with your abdominals tight.

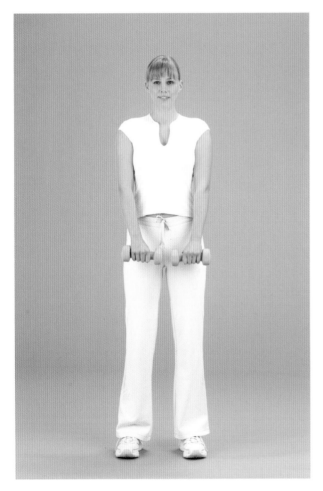

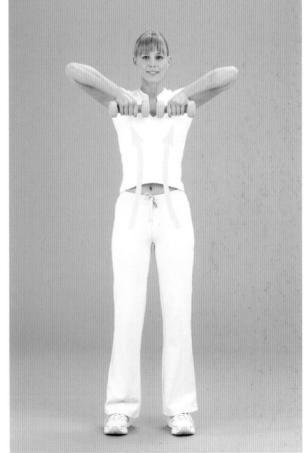

1 Stand with your feet hip-width apart and a dumb-bell in each hand in front of your body, with your hands close together.

2 Bend the elbows and lift the weights until they are at chest height. Your elbows should be slightly above your shoulders and your wrists should be straight. Lower the weights back down to the starting position. Aim for 16 lifts.

shoulder SHRUG

The aim of this exercise is to **develop the trapezius muscle** that runs from the neck down the back.

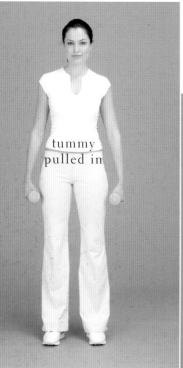

tummy
pulled in

1 Stand with your feet hip-width apart and your arms by your sides. Hold a dumb-bell in each hand.

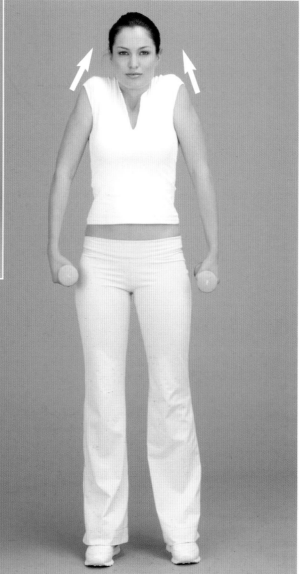

2 Lift your shoulders up to the ears and then lower them, keeping the arms straight at all times. Repeat. Aim for 16 shrugs.

TRAINER TIPS

Press the shoulders back and down after each lift.

Pull in your abdominal muscles and hold them tight during the exercise.

bent-over ROW

This exercise works the latissimus dorsi muscle of the back, stretching from the armpit to the gluteals. Working this muscle will help to **define and shape the back**.

1 Step forward on the right foot and bend the right knee, bringing the shoulders over the right foot. Hold a dumb-bell in the left hand and down by your left side. Your right hand should rest on your right thigh and your back should be straight.

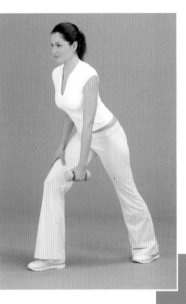

TRAINER TIPS

Keep the abdominal muscles tight and draw the belly button back to the spine throughout.

This exercise can be performed with your knee resting on a bench to aid stability.

2 Pull up the weight in your left hand, bending the elbow, keeping it away from the body and the wrist straight. The weight should come up past your hip, towards your chest, and your back should be kept flat. The left shoulder blade should be squeezed in towards the spine. Return the weight to the starting position, then repeat on the other side. Aim for 16 lifts.

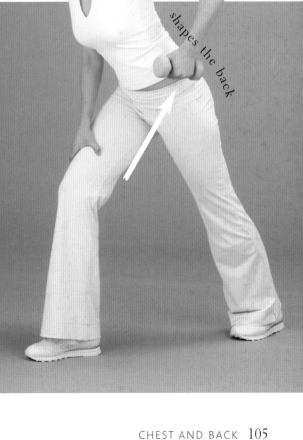

shapes the back

arm PRESS-UP

This press-up is **great for the chest**, but works other muscles too, such as those of the back, abdominals, shoulders and legs. There are a variety of ways to perform it.

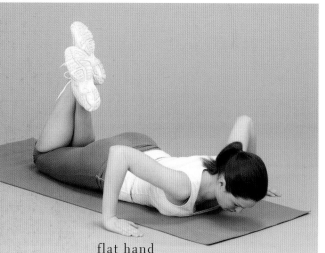

flat hand

1 Lie face down on the mat, with your ankles crossed and your hands on each side of your chest, slightly wider than shoulder-width apart.

2 Press your body up on to your knees, keeping your back and neck in a straight line by using your arms. Your chin should be relaxed and down. Pull in your abdominals and keep your belly button drawn up to your spine.

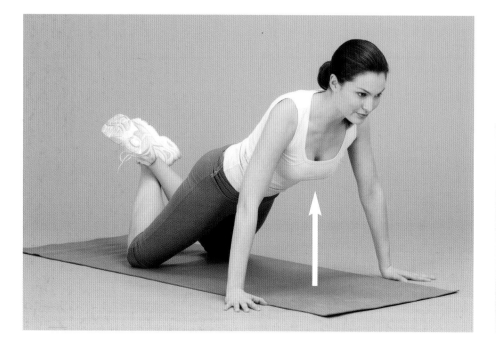

TRAINER TIP

Do not let your hips lift too high in the advanced version of the press-up.

3 Lower back towards your mat by bending your elbows, but do not let your chest touch the mat. As you near it with your chest, push yourself back up. Aim for 20 press-ups.

REALLY WORK IT!

To make this exercise harder, lie face down as before, but with your legs fully extended and feet slightly apart. Turn your toes under so that you are resting on them. Push yourself up using your hands, and rest on your toes. Your body should be in a straight line from your feet to your shoulders.

Lower your body towards the floor and, just before reaching the mat, push back up. Aim for 20 press-ups.

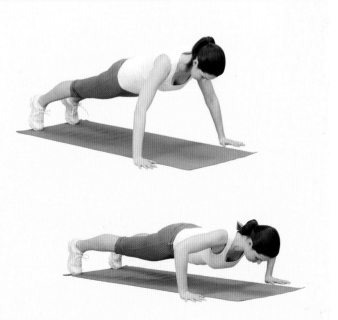

back EXTENSION

Excellent for working the back, this exercise strengthens the core muscles and helps improve posture.

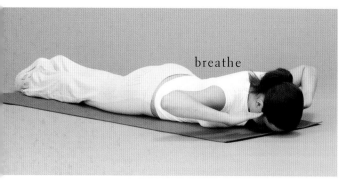

breathe

1 Lie face down on the mat, with your hands on each side of your head, and your legs fully extended.

2 Breathe out as you lift your head and chest off the mat, keeping your hips and pubic bone on the floor and your head and neck in alignment.

TRAINER TIP

Make sure you get your breathing right, as this will help you as you lift.

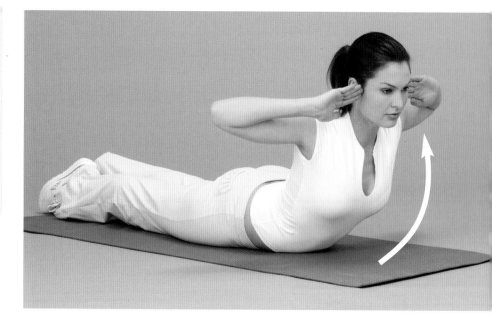

3 Breathe in as you lower yourself back to the ground. Aim for 8–12 lifts.

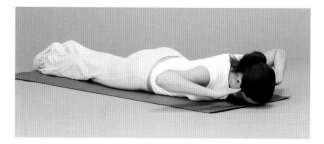

cobra LIFT

This is a good exercise for **toning the back** extensor muscles.

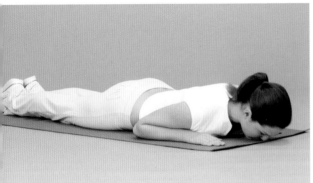

1 Lie face down on your mat, with your hands by your shoulders and your elbows bent.

TRAINER TIP

Rotate your feet outwards on the floor, as this helps to support your lower back. You will be able to place less weight in your hands as your back lengthens.

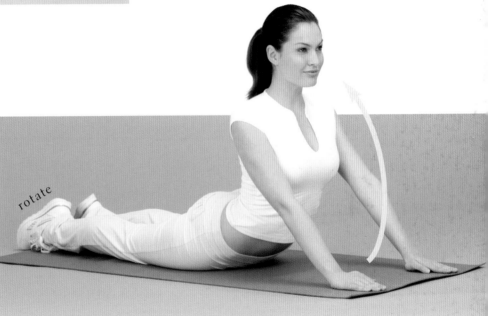

rotate

2 Breathe out as you slowly lift your head and chest off the mat, pressing your weight on to your hands and straightening your arms. Do not worry if you can not straighten your elbows to start with. Keep your neck in line and tighten your abdominal muscles. Hold for a count of two. Breathe in as you lower your chest to the floor. Then lift and repeat again. Aim for ten lifts.

leg LIFT for back

This leg lift will help to strengthen the lower back.

1 Lie on your stomach, with your hands under your forehead and your legs straight.

TRAINER TIP

By keeping your hips on the mat, you will work the lower back more effectively.

2 Pull up your abdominal muscles and lift your right leg straight off the mat, as high as you can. Hold for a count of two and then lower. Repeat on the left leg, making sure you do not lift your hips off the mat. Aim for 16 lifts.

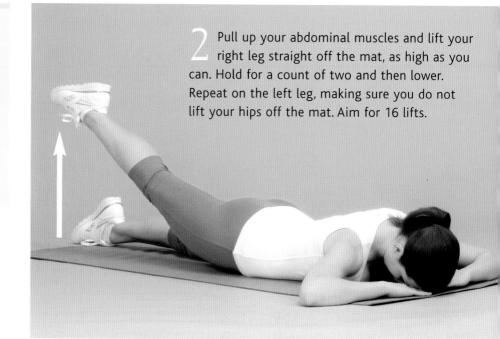

superman LIFT

This lift also really helps to **tone the** muscles of the lower back.

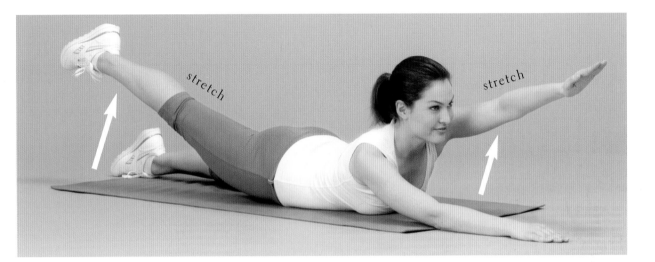

stretch   *stretch*

1 Lie face down on the mat, with your hands outstretched in front of you so that they are parallel to the floor, palms facing down. Lift your left arm, right leg and chest, head and shoulders off the mat. You are now stretching in opposite directions. Hold for a count of two and lower back down. Repeat with your right arm and left leg.

TRAINER TIPS

Breathe evenly throughout the exercise, even when holding the lifts.

Pull in the abdominals as you lift, and pull your shoulder blades down and back at the same time.

REALLY WORK IT!

Then lift your arms, head, chest and both legs off the mat and hold for a count of two. Avoid arching the neck. Lower and repeat. Aim for 16 lifts.

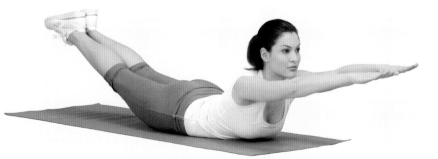

front RAISE

Another useful exercise for **working** the chest.

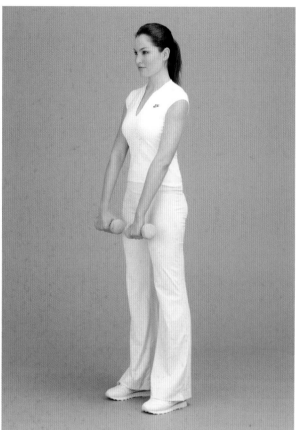
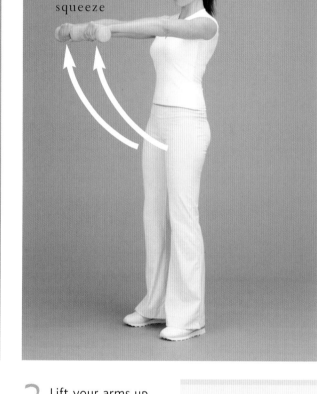

squeeze

1 Stand with your feet hip-width apart and a weight in each hand. Your arms should be held in front of your body, resting just in front of your thighs.

2 Lift your arms up to shoulder level, squeeze the weights in each hand as you lift, with the palms facing down to the floor. Lower back down and repeat. Aim for 16 raises.

TRAINER TIPS

Ensure that you have tightened your abdominal muscles before you lift.

Keep your back straight.

ROLL down

This roll down will help to stretch out the spine and enable you to engage your core muscles as your body moves.

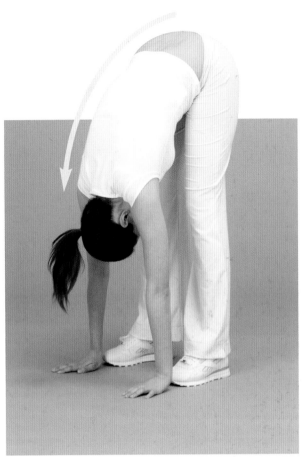

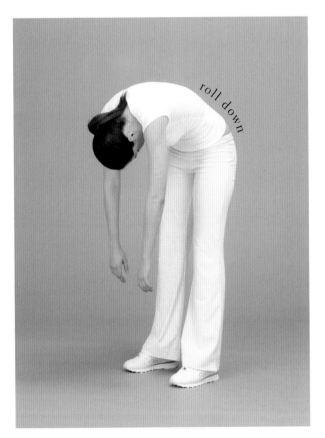

roll down

1 Stand straight and tall with your legs hip-width apart. Bend your knees a little and relax your shoulders. Breathe out, drawing your belly button into your spine, then start to roll downwards by bringing your chin to your chest, down through your neck, upper back and lower back. Your shoulders will round forwards as you begin to roll down. If you feel uncomfortable on the way down, increase the bend in your knees.

2 Aim to take your hands to the floor. Only roll down as far as you comfortably can. Once down there, breathe in and out for four slow breaths, then slowly start to roll back up. Repeat twice.

TRAINER TIPS

Perform the exercise slowly so your spine has time to lengthen and stretch.

You may find that your hamstrings (at the back of your legs) are tight to begin with, but these will stretch and lengthen in time.

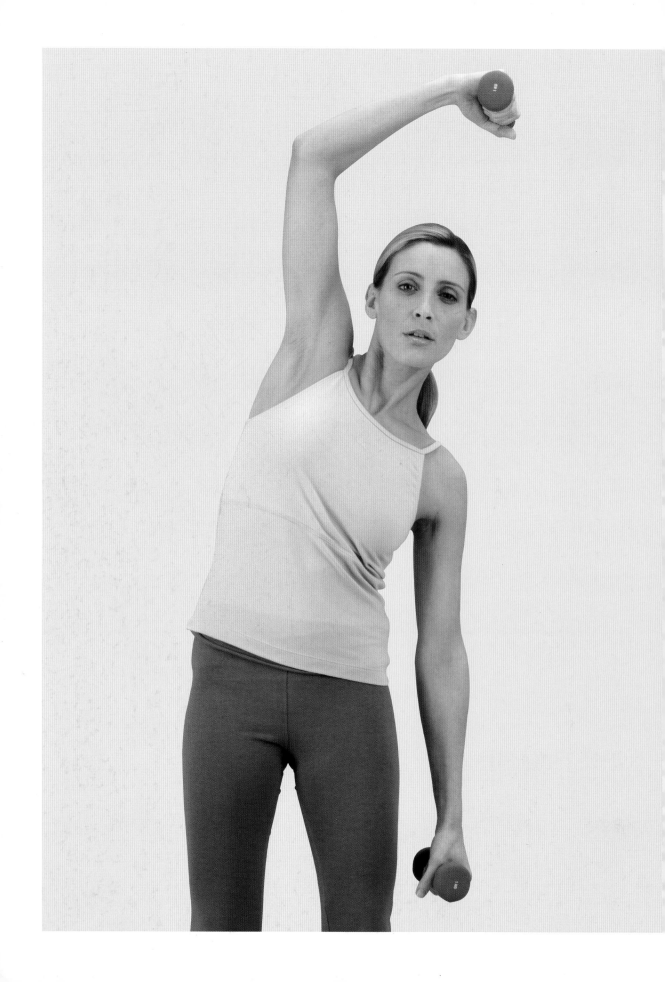

The Four-Week Plan

For each of the four one-week plans, start your session with a warm up of five minutes of aerobic exercise. Choose from one of the following activities – jogging on the spot, brisk walking, bouncing on a mini-trampoline, cycling, rowing or swimming – and remember to start slowly and build up, so that you warm up the muscles gradually. Follow with the stretches given on pages 26–27. At the end of each session, finish with the cool-down stretches described on pages 28–29.

Week 1

On each day complete the two 10-minute routines suggested, focusing on different areas of the body.

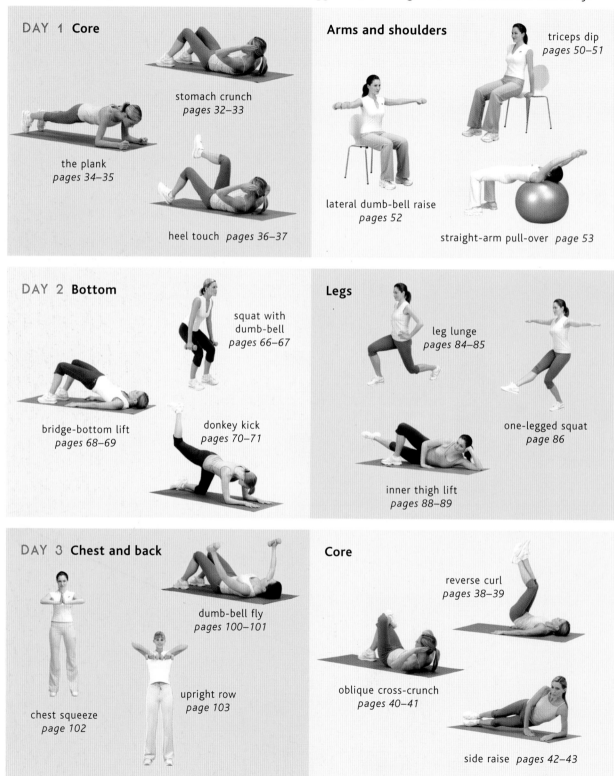

DAY 1 **Core**

stomach crunch
pages 32–33

the plank
pages 34–35

heel touch *pages 36–37*

Arms and shoulders

triceps dip
pages 50–51

lateral dumb-bell raise
pages 52

straight-arm pull-over *page 53*

DAY 2 **Bottom**

squat with
dumb-bell
pages 66–67

bridge-bottom lift
pages 68–69

donkey kick
pages 70–71

Legs

leg lunge
pages 84–85

one-legged squat
page 86

inner thigh lift
pages 88–89

DAY 3 **Chest and back**

dumb-bell fly
pages 100–101

upright row
page 103

chest squeeze
page 102

Core

reverse curl
pages 38–39

oblique cross-crunch
pages 40–41

side raise *pages 42–43*

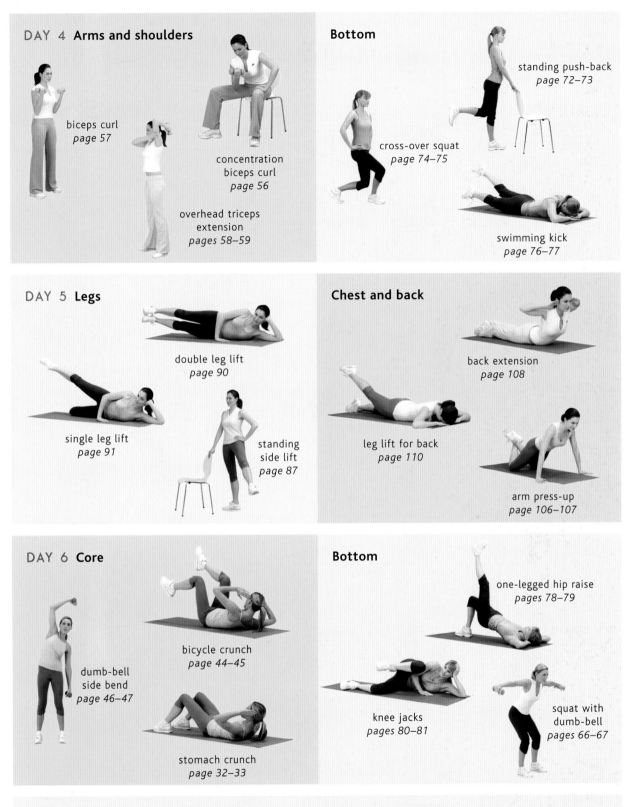

DAY 4 Arms and shoulders

biceps curl
page 57

concentration
biceps curl
page 56

overhead triceps
extension
pages 58–59

Bottom

standing push-back
page 72–73

cross-over squat
page 74–75

swimming kick
page 76–77

DAY 5 Legs

double leg lift
page 90

single leg lift
page 91

standing
side lift
page 87

Chest and back

back extension
page 108

leg lift for back
page 110

arm press-up
page 106–107

DAY 6 Core

dumb-bell
side bend
page 46–47

bicycle crunch
page 44–45

stomach crunch
page 32–33

Bottom

one-legged hip raise
pages 78–79

knee jacks
pages 80–81

squat with
dumb-bell
pages 66–67

DAY 7 REST DAY

Week 2

On each day complete the two 10-minute routines suggested, focusing on different areas of the body.

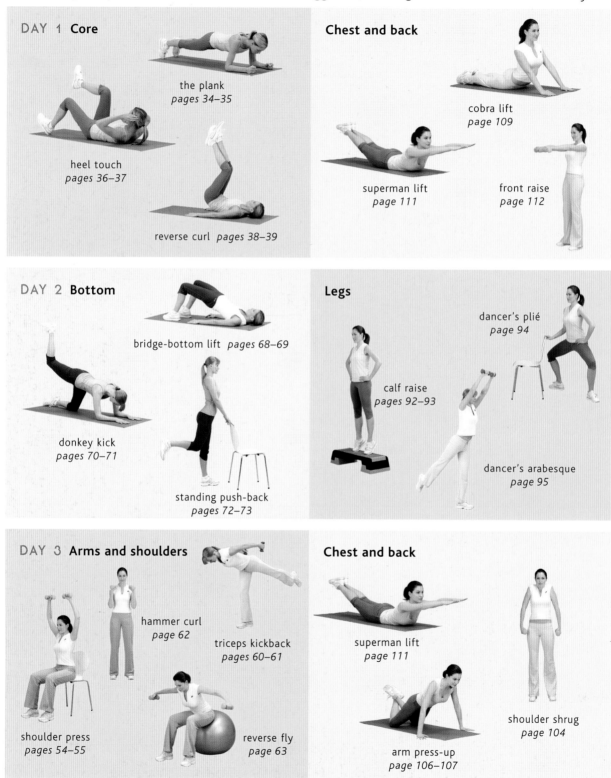

DAY 1 **Core**

the plank
pages 34–35

heel touch
pages 36–37

reverse curl pages 38–39

Chest and back

cobra lift
page 109

superman lift
page 111

front raise
page 112

DAY 2 **Bottom**

bridge-bottom lift pages 68–69

donkey kick
pages 70–71

standing push-back
pages 72–73

Legs

dancer's plié
page 94

calf raise
pages 92–93

dancer's arabesque
page 95

DAY 3 **Arms and shoulders**

hammer curl
page 62

triceps kickback
pages 60–61

shoulder press
pages 54–55

reverse fly
page 63

Chest and back

superman lift
page 111

arm press-up
page 106–107

shoulder shrug
page 104

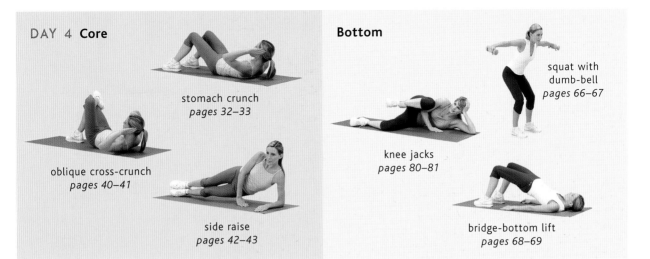

DAY 4 Core

stomach crunch
pages 32–33

oblique cross-crunch
pages 40–41

side raise
pages 42–43

Bottom

squat with
dumb-bell
pages 66–67

knee jacks
pages 80–81

bridge-bottom lift
pages 68–69

DAY 5 REST DAY

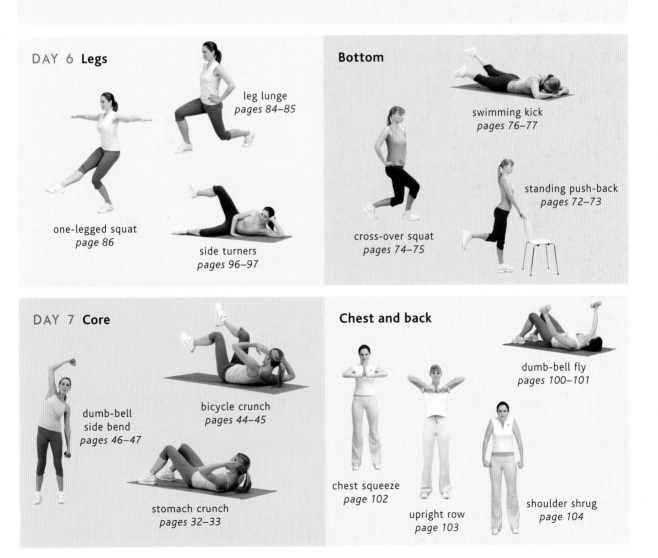

DAY 6 Legs

leg lunge
pages 84–85

one-legged squat
page 86

side turners
pages 96–97

Bottom

swimming kick
pages 76–77

standing push-back
pages 72–73

cross-over squat
pages 74–75

DAY 7 Core

dumb-bell
side bend
pages 46–47

bicycle crunch
pages 44–45

stomach crunch
pages 32–33

Chest and back

dumb-bell fly
pages 100–101

chest squeeze
page 102

upright row
page 103

shoulder shrug
page 104

Week 3

On each day complete the three 10-minute routines suggested, focusing on different areas of the body.

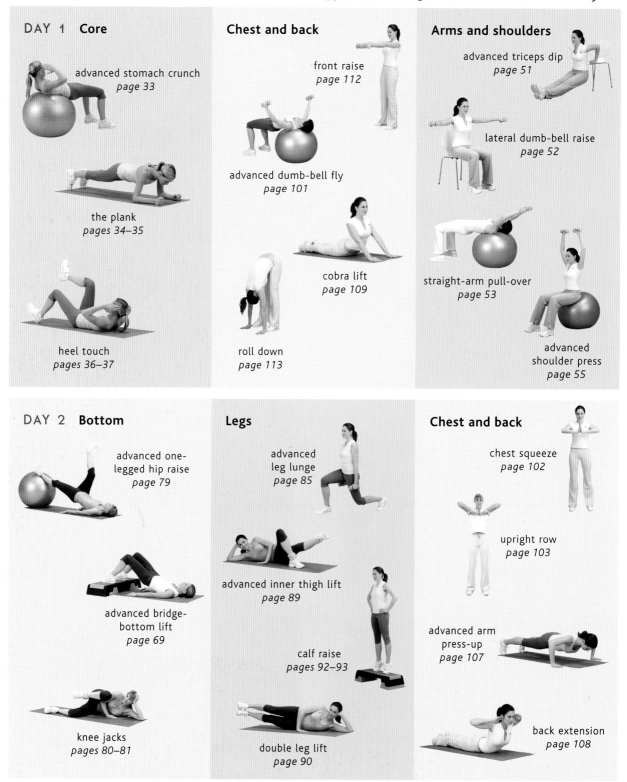

DAY 1 **Core**

advanced stomach crunch
page 33

the plank
pages 34–35

heel touch
pages 36–37

Chest and back

front raise
page 112

advanced dumb-bell fly
page 101

cobra lift
page 109

roll down
page 113

Arms and shoulders

advanced triceps dip
page 51

lateral dumb-bell raise
page 52

straight-arm pull-over
page 53

advanced shoulder press
page 55

DAY 2 **Bottom**

advanced one-legged hip raise
page 79

advanced bridge-bottom lift
page 69

knee jacks
pages 80–81

Legs

advanced leg lunge
page 85

advanced inner thigh lift
page 89

calf raise
pages 92–93

double leg lift
page 90

Chest and back

chest squeeze
page 102

upright row
page 103

advanced arm press-up
page 107

back extension
page 108

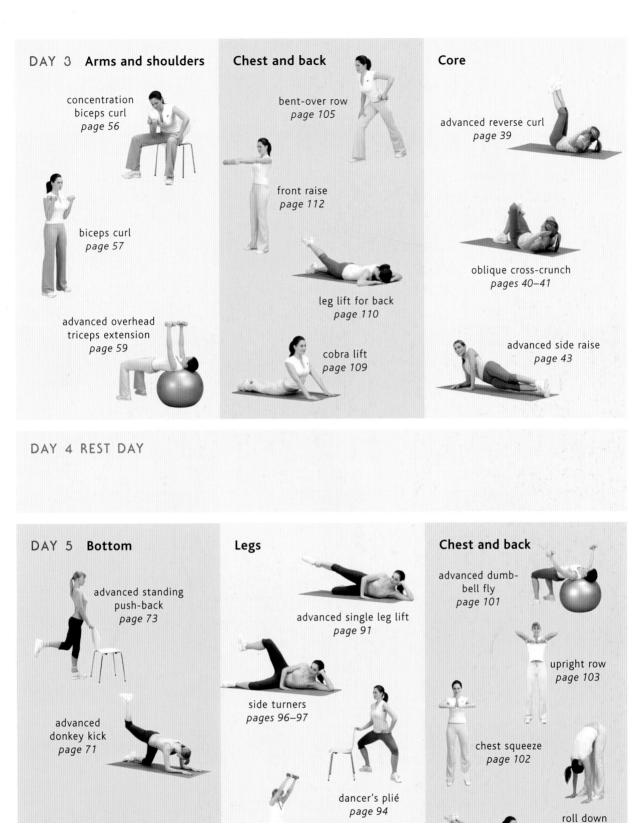

DAY 3   Arms and shoulders

concentration
biceps curl
page 56

biceps curl
page 57

advanced overhead
triceps extension
page 59

Chest and back

bent-over row
page 105

front raise
page 112

leg lift for back
page 110

cobra lift
page 109

Core

advanced reverse curl
page 39

oblique cross-crunch
pages 40–41

advanced side raise
page 43

DAY 4 REST DAY

DAY 5   Bottom

advanced standing
push-back
page 73

advanced
donkey kick
page 71

swimming kick
pages 76–77

Legs

advanced single leg lift
page 91

side turners
pages 96–97

dancer's plié
page 94

dancer's arabesque
page 95

Chest and back

advanced dumb-
bell fly
page 101

upright row
page 103

chest squeeze
page 102

roll down
page 113

superman lift
page 111

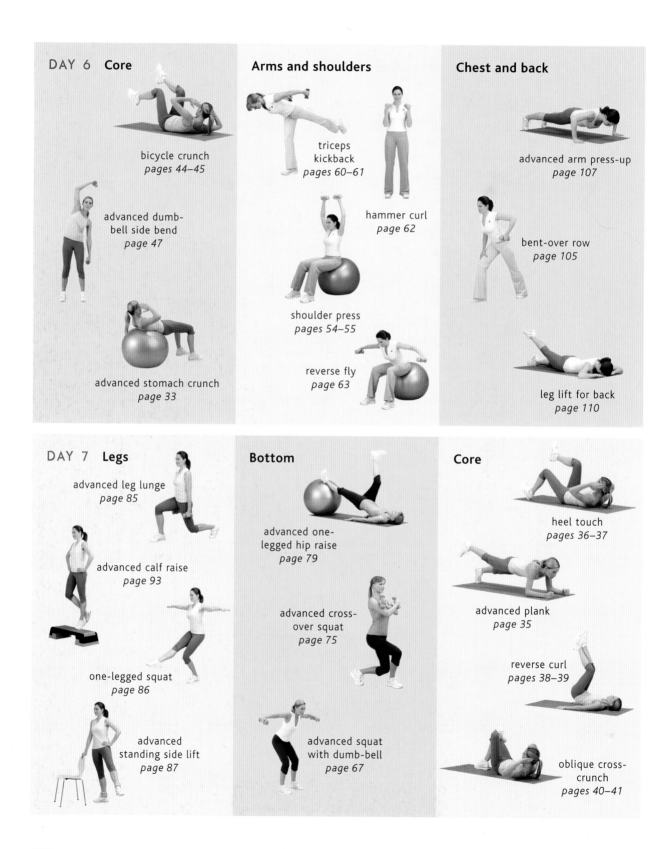

DAY 6 Core

bicycle crunch
pages 44–45

advanced dumb-
bell side bend
page 47

advanced stomach crunch
page 33

Arms and shoulders

triceps
kickback
pages 60–61

hammer curl
page 62

shoulder press
pages 54–55

reverse fly
page 63

Chest and back

advanced arm press-up
page 107

bent-over row
page 105

leg lift for back
page 110

DAY 7 Legs

advanced leg lunge
page 85

advanced calf raise
page 93

one-legged squat
page 86

advanced
standing side lift
page 87

Bottom

advanced one-
legged hip raise
page 79

advanced cross-
over squat
page 75

advanced squat
with dumb-bell
page 67

Core

heel touch
pages 36–37

advanced plank
page 35

reverse curl
pages 38–39

oblique cross-
crunch
pages 40–41

Week 4

On each day complete the three 10-minute routines suggested, focusing on different areas of the body.

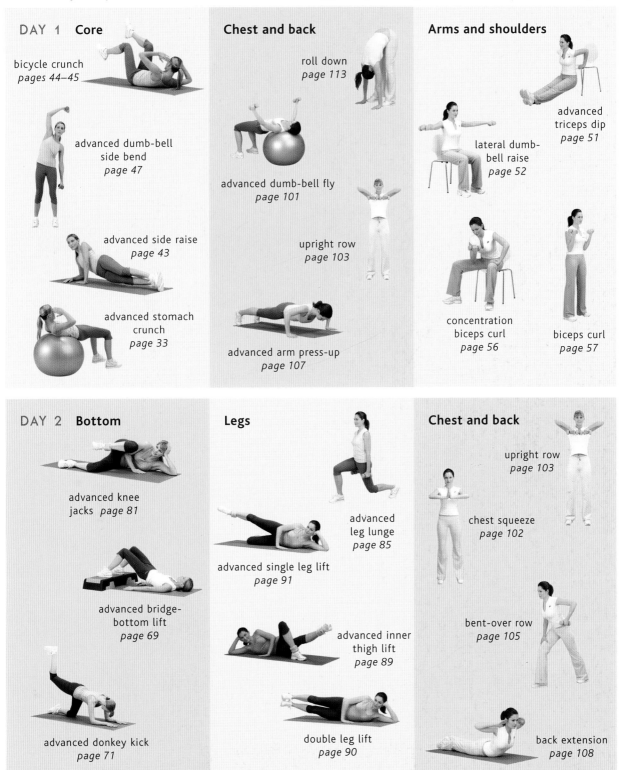

DAY 1 **Core**

bicycle crunch
pages 44–45

advanced dumb-bell
side bend
page 47

advanced side raise
page 43

advanced stomach
crunch
page 33

Chest and back

roll down
page 113

advanced dumb-bell fly
page 101

upright row
page 103

advanced arm press-up
page 107

Arms and shoulders

advanced
triceps dip
page 51

lateral dumb-
bell raise
page 52

concentration
biceps curl
page 56

biceps curl
page 57

DAY 2 **Bottom**

advanced knee
jacks *page 81*

advanced bridge-
bottom lift
page 69

advanced donkey kick
page 71

Legs

advanced
leg lunge
page 85

advanced single leg lift
page 91

advanced inner
thigh lift
page 89

double leg lift
page 90

Chest and back

upright row
page 103

chest squeeze
page 102

bent-over row
page 105

back extension
page 108

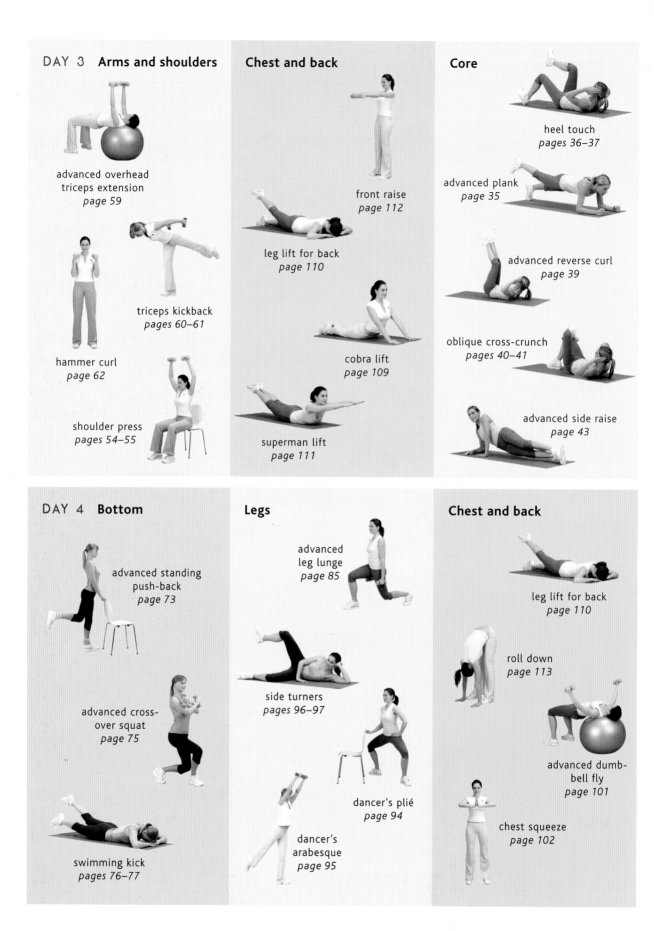

DAY 3 Arms and shoulders

advanced overhead
triceps extension
page 59

triceps kickback
pages 60–61

hammer curl
page 62

shoulder press
pages 54–55

Chest and back

front raise
page 112

leg lift for back
page 110

cobra lift
page 109

superman lift
page 111

Core

heel touch
pages 36–37

advanced plank
page 35

advanced reverse curl
page 39

oblique cross-crunch
pages 40–41

advanced side raise
page 43

DAY 4 Bottom

advanced standing
push-back
page 73

advanced cross-
over squat
page 75

swimming kick
pages 76–77

Legs

advanced
leg lunge
page 85

side turners
pages 96–97

dancer's plié
page 94

dancer's
arabesque
page 95

Chest and back

leg lift for back
page 110

roll down
page 113

advanced dumb-
bell fly
page 101

chest squeeze
page 102

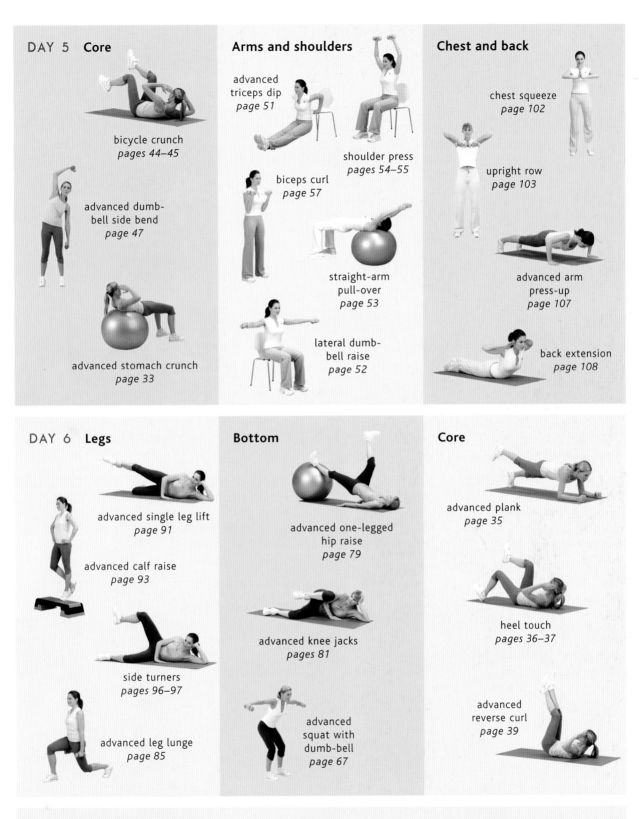

DAY 5 Core

bicycle crunch
pages 44–45

advanced dumb-bell side bend
page 47

advanced stomach crunch
page 33

Arms and shoulders

advanced triceps dip
page 51

biceps curl
page 57

shoulder press
pages 54–55

straight-arm pull-over
page 53

lateral dumb-bell raise
page 52

Chest and back

chest squeeze
page 102

upright row
page 103

advanced arm press-up
page 107

back extension
page 108

DAY 6 Legs

advanced single leg lift
page 91

advanced calf raise
page 93

side turners
pages 96–97

advanced leg lunge
page 85

Bottom

advanced one-legged hip raise
page 79

advanced knee jacks
pages 81

advanced squat with dumb-bell
page 67

Core

advanced plank
page 35

heel touch
pages 36–37

advanced reverse curl
page 39

DAY 7 REST DAY

Index

Acknowledgments

Author acknowledgements
I would like to thank all my clients, past and present, for
their contributions and support – keep at it and the
results will show for themselves. To Jane and her team
at Hamlyn, Ruth and Penny for smiling the whole time
through the photo shoot – we got there in the end.
Many thanks. To Mark, Alex and Harrison, and of course
mum and dad, for their love and support.

Special photography
© Octopus Publishing Group/Mike Prior

Other photography
Octopus Publishing Group Limited/Janine Hosegood 12,
13, 15; /Mike Prior 9, 21; /Peter Pugh-Cook 19, 19, 22;
/Russell Sadur 10, 11.
PhotoDisc 14.

Executive editor: Jane MacIntosh
Project editor: Ruth Wiseall
Executive art editor: Penny Stock
Designer: Geoff Borin
Picture researcher: Ciaran O'Reilly
Production controller: Martin Croshaw